# Research and Research Methods for Youth Practitioners

Rigorous research is crucial to effective work with young people, and increasingly youth practitioners need to be able to develop, review and evidence their work using a variety of research and assessment tools. This text equips students and practitioners with a thorough understanding of research design, practice and dissemination, as well as approaches to evidence-based practice.

A clear practice framework informs the book, outlining the significance of research to youth work, especially in relation to designing and developing services for young people. *Research and Research Methods for Youth Practitioners*:

- analyses the practitioner-researcher role
- explores the ethical context of research in youth work
- offers a thorough analysis of key methodological questions in research in practice
- provides a guide to data collection and analysis
- presents five principal research strategies for youth work: ethnographic work and visual methods; interviewing and evaluation; surveys and evaluation; the use of secondary data and documentary analysis; and researching virtual and online settings
- discusses the implications of research for work with young people as well as its dissemination.

Written by experienced researchers and practitioner-researchers, each chapter in this accessible textbook includes an overview, a critical discussion of the pros and cons of the particular method or approach, a case study, a practice-based task, a summary and suggestions for further reading. This textbook is invaluable for student and practising youth workers. It is also a useful reference for other practitioners working with young people.

**Simon Bradford** is Reader in Social Sciences in the School of Health Sciences and Social Care at Brunel University, UK.

**Fin Cullen** is Lecturer in Youth and Community Studies in the School of Health Sciences and Social Care at Brunel University, UK.

# Research and Research Methods for Youth Practitioners

## Edited by Simon Bradford and Fin Cullen

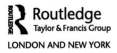

Routledge
Taylor & Francis Group

LONDON AND NEW YORK

First published 2012
by Routledge
2 Park Square, Milton Park, Abingdon, Oxon OX14 4RN

Simultaneously published in the USA and Canada
by Routledge
711 Third Avenue, New York, NY 10017

*Routledge is an imprint of the Taylor & Francis Group, an informa business*

*British Library Cataloguing in Publication Data*
A catalogue record for this book is available from the British Library

*Library of Congress Cataloging in Publication Data*
Research and research methods for youth practitioners / edited by Simon Bradford and Fin Cullen.
    p. cm.
1. Social work with youth. 2. Youth workers. 3. Social sciences—Research. I. Bradford, Simon. II. Cullen, Fin.
HV1421.R458 2012
362.7—dc22                                          2011014005

ISBN: 978-0-415-57085-5 (hbk)
ISBN: 978-0-415-57103-6 (pbk)
ISBN: 978-0-203-80257-1 (ebk)

Typeset in Sabon
by Keystroke, Station Road, Codsall, Wolverhampton

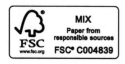
MIX
Paper from
responsible sources
FSC www.fsc.org  FSC® C004839

Printed and bound in Great Britain by
TJ International Ltd, Padstow, Cornwall

This book is dedicated to the memory of Dr Michael Lewis Day,
friend and teacher, 20 February 1940–3 March 2010.

# Contents

# Contributors

**Alexandra Allan** is Lecturer in Education, Childhood and Youth Studies in the School of Education, Exeter University. Alexandra's Ph.D. focused on young girls' constructions of femininity. Her recent research has focused on young women's perceptions of risk. Both of these projects have utilised ethnographic and visual methods.

**Pam Alldred** lectures in the Centre for Youth Work Studies at Brunel University. She writes and teaches about the politics of research in the social sciences and education, and the dilemmas of representing children and young people. She has contributed to several feminist research methods books and to the SIMREF feminist research methodology international school.

**John Barker** is a geographer and Lecturer in the Social Work Division at Brunel University. John's research and teaching specialises in different aspects of children's and young people's lives, including childcare, play, education, travel and access to services and activities, as well as methodological debates surrounding researching children, childhood and youth.

**Albert Bell** is Head of the Department for Youth and Community Studies at the University of Malta. He is also presently chair of the Foundation of Education Services (FES) and of the National Domestic Violence Commission's Research and Data Collection Subcommittee. His research interests include youth and music subcultures, juvenile justice and youth deviance.

**Judith Bessant** is Professor of Youth Studies and Sociology at Royal Melbourne Institute of Technology University, Australia. She has worked for government and non-government organisations in Australia and internationally to develop policy. She has also published widely in the areas of sociology, policy, youth studies, education, social theory and policy.

**Simon Bradford** is Reader in Social Sciences in the School of Health Sciences and Social Care at Brunel University. His research interests include youth and youth cultures, social policy as it affects young people and communities, and professionalisation and professional identities of those who work with young people. He is Director of the Centre for Youth Work Studies at Brunel University.

**Marilyn Clark** received her doctorate from the University of Sheffield and is Senior Lecturer with the Department of Youth and Community Studies at the University of Malta. Marilyn's main research interests are criminal and addictive careers. She chairs the National Commission for the Abuse of Drugs, Alcohol and Other Dependencies and has published both in Malta and overseas.

**Clare Choak** has eight years' experience researching young people's lives, three of which were spent conducting ethnographic research with young women in deprived areas, focusing on their engagement with youth work interventions. She is also Senior Lecturer in Research Methods and Research Fellow at the University of Greenwich. Her research interests include working class young women, gang involved young people, and offending behaviour.

**Nic Crowe** is a qualified teacher, youth and community worker and Fellow of the Higher Education Academy. He is currently Lecturer in Education at Brunel University. His Ph.D. thesis focused on young people's use of the internet for gaming, and looked particularly at virtual identities, virtual communities and their culture(s).

**Fin Cullen** is Lecturer in Youth and Community Studies in the School of Health Sciences and Social Care at Brunel University. Since 1997, Fin has been involved in youth work and research projects across the UK. Her research interests include participatory action research, youth sexualities, girls' drinking cultures, visual methods and youth geographies.

**Rys Farthing** is currently completing her doctorate in social policy at Oxford University. She has previously taught youth work at universities in Australia and the UK. Outside of academia, she has worked with a number of child rights based NGOs analysing public policy.

**Laura Green** is a Ph.D. student and Lecturer in Youth and Community Studies at Brunel University. She is also a professionally qualified youth worker. Laura uses contemporary, interactive research methods that are child/young person friendly and aims to encourage young people to become research partners and collaborate in research design.

**Geeta Ludhra** is Lecturer in Education at Brunel University where she teaches on the Initial Teacher Education programme. Her background is in primary teaching and she has worked in various teaching, management and advisory roles within London schools. Her current doctoral research focuses on the topic of cultural identities of South Asian young women.

**Chrissie Rogers** is Reader in Education at Anglia Ruskin University. Her main interests are related to intellectual disability, 'inclusive' education, mothering, intimacy, disability theory and qualitative research methods. Chrissie is the author of *Parenting and Inclusive Education* and she has recently joined the editorial board of the *British Journal of Sociology of Education*.

**Stan Tucker** is Professor Emeritus at Newman University College in Birmingham. He has researched and published widely in the areas of education and social policy. His recent co-edited book *Early Childhoods in a Changing World* reflects his interest in exploring the life stories of children and young people.

# Acknowledgements

We wish to acknowledge the practical help, support and patience offered by many people during the editing and writing of the book. We particularly appreciate the support and involvement of Laura Green, Michael Whelan and everyone involved in the Centre for Youth Work Studies at Brunel University.

Thanks are also due to all the contributors, and past and present students at CYWS, who are always keen to be inspired and to inspire, discuss and debate the issues raised in this book.

Fin warmly thanks old and new youth work colleagues – particularly Rich Campbell and the youth café bus team – for their commitment and our debates about the purpose, direction and 'success' of contemporary youth work.

Thanks to everyone who gave us advice on the book. Any errors are, of course, our own.

Finally, we both acknowledge the support of our families and friends. Fin is particularly grateful for the support of her family, and her grandmother, Jean Cullen, who passed away during the final editing of the book.

# Introduction

Simon Bradford and Fin Cullen

The contemporary landscape presents youth practitioners (and, more importantly perhaps, *young people*) with enormous challenges. Recent policy shifts (Every Child Matters and Aiming High for Young People, for example, in the UK) have demanded a new reflexivity on the part of youth professionals, and have led to new kinds of services for children and young people. During the last decade, the concept of professionalism in the public services has been carefully scrutinised, and professionals across Europe and elsewhere have become increasingly subject to regimes of audit and performativity. More recent political changes in the UK and other countries (including aspirations for a 'smaller state' and increased reliance on voluntary and third sectors), if implemented, will shift the configuration and governance of public services, leading to radically altered provision for young people and communities. For example, the inception of the 'Big Society' discourse from the coalition government in the UK will alter the provision and types of services available to young people. Changing political priorities will also shape future provision, and we can expect much more attention to be given to services that target very specific groups and geographical locations. In this context it will be important for managers and practitioners to be able to undertake and draw on good research to provide evidence for success in their work.

Macro political and economic changes in the post-recessionary world are transforming the social and material settings in which young people grow up. New (and reworked) definitions and discourses of youth need will shape the services that emerge or develop over the next few years. Many young people will experience increased disadvantage and their aspirations are likely to be tested and sometimes dashed. In such circumstances, youth practitioners will be important sources of support. Crucially, service providers in the voluntary and third sectors (some of which may have limited experience in the field) and professionals will have to be able to acquire accurate and robust knowledge of the circumstances of young people and their communities. This will be necessary to ensure that services are relevant and appropriate for young people, but also to be able to argue cases for support from funders. The importance of careful planning, data collection and analysis to practitioners' and service managers' work (practice and policy development) is central to this book's overall approach.

The book starts from the conviction that effective professional intervention and development with young people and communities can be made only on the basis of carefully planned and thoughtful research (although well-designed organisations, skilful practice and competent managers are also vital). Good research provides necessary knowledge and insight into the circumstances that young people face in their daily lives and the basis upon which policy-makers and professionals can make good judgements about interventions. To be an effective and critical youth practitioner thus necessitates an engagement with and development of analytic and research-based knowledge and skills. This book aims to support this.

The book is aimed at practitioners and managers in youth practice (youth work and related settings of work with young people and communities) and students undertaking courses of qualifying professional education for work with young people at either undergraduate or master's level. Because each chapter includes case studies, practice-based tasks and suggestions for further reading, the book can be used as a source for teaching and learning in both formal and informal settings.

The aim is to provide help to practitioner-researchers and managers in developing their capacity in undertaking effective research in their work settings. The book identifies key methodological questions in practitioner-research, provides a guide to data collection and analysis, and offers a thorough discussion of the presentation of research findings and the contexts in which that might occur.

The often contested, complex and attenuated relationship between research, policy and practice is identified, but a clear practice framework informs each chapter. This emphasises youth work's value stance and, in particular, it raises important questions about young people's participation in research.

## Organisation of the book

The contributors to this book are all active researchers, educators and practitioners in the fields of youth and education. As practitioners, they have participated in a range of research projects, and they have first-hand experience of the complex challenges of 'doing research' in youth practice contexts.

In the opening chapter, Fin Cullen, Simon Bradford and Laura Green ask what research is for, and outline the possible tensions and conflicts that can arise when entering the field as a practitioner *and* researcher. The practitioner-researcher role is explored in some detail. Chapter 1 also investigates and outlines Participatory Action Research (PAR), and discusses how research might directly influence and shape both policy and practice. Finally, it touches on questions of research, power and ethics.

Stan Tucker, in Chapter 2, offers a framework for designing and developing a research project. Tucker emphasises the importance of understanding research as a process in which a number of linked stages (including defining a problem, choosing a methodology, collecting, analysing and interpreting data) have to be planned and worked through by the practitioner-researcher in order to produce good-quality research. In particular, Chapter 2 stresses the importance of identifying a clear research question at the outset of the research process. Without this, good research is unlikely to be possible.

In Chapter 3, Chrissie Rogers and Geeta Ludhra consider the nature and significance of research ethics and relate this to questions of social difference, consent, 'voice' and participation. The chapter draws attention to a range of dilemmas that are likely to be faced by the practitioner-researcher in research with young people and communities. Rogers and Ludhra problematise the notion of *informed consent* and interrogate its meaning for practitioner-researchers. They suggest that informed consent should reflect a real commitment to young people's participation and inclusion in the research process from the planning stages through to dissemination of the research findings. Where young people are intensively involved, they suggest, research that offers good research-based accounts of young people's lives (sometimes including troubled and difficult aspects of these) is possible.

Alexandra Allan looks at ethnography and the use of visual methods of data collection in Chapter 4. Allan highlights the value of ethnographic research and the use of visual methods in researching the detailed cultural dimensions of young people's daily lives. Ethnography's capacity to collect rich data makes it ideal for understanding young people's cultural practices and the social relations in which these are structured. Visual methods have become an important means of collecting data on young people and youth cultures, and they are especially useful in involving young people themselves.

In Chapter 5, Clare Choak suggests that contemporary society has become saturated by interviews and interviewing (through television and the media generally) and that people are routinely familiar with the interview as a data collection tool. Interviews – and asking questions – have become a principal means for practitioner-researchers to collect data. Choak outlines different kinds of interviews and discusses how the data that are generated by these might be used to inform youth practice.

Marilyn Clark and Albert Bell consider quantitative research methodologies in Chapter 6. They emphasise the importance of rigour in quantitative research design, identify the strengths and limitations of quantitative methodologies in practitioner research, and dispel some of the misunderstandings and myths that surround them. They show that quantitative surveys are an important means of acquiring potentially large quantities of data that can provide important insights into young people's views. Clark and Bell identify a number of important ethical considerations that practitioner-researchers should take into account in quantitative studies.

In Chapter 7, John Barker and Pam Alldred discuss the use of documentary evidence and secondary data. They point to the vast array of documents that characterise late modern societies and suggest that these provide the practitioner-researcher with potentially important data sources. Secondary sources – government reports, historical documents or official records, for example – contain large quantities of data that provide insights into young people's lives, and a number of substantive secondary sources relevant to youth practitioner-researchers are identified. Most importantly, Barker and Alldred indicate that practitioner-researchers should treat these documentary and secondary data sources critically. As they point out, documents are socially constructed and invariably reflect the positions and power of those producing them.

In Chapter 8, Nic Crowe discusses the possibilities for practitioner-researchers to collect data from online and virtual sources. Crowe argues that virtual worlds and online gaming arenas (such as *Second Life* and *World of Warcraft*) have become important leisure-time settings in which young people construct aspects of their social identities. Virtual ethnography, Crowe suggests, should be seen as a source of interesting and important data on youth cultures. This is both similar to and different from ethnography undertaken in the material everyday world, and Crowe considers some of the arguments put forward by Allan in Chapter 4 in relation to virtuality. The chapter identifies some key research strategies for collecting data in virtual settings.

For many practitioner-researchers there is also a clear political need to let policy-makers, funders, other scholars, managers, young people and the wider public know about their research findings. The processes and challenges involved in the dissemination of research are considered in Chapter 9. Here, Judith Bessant and Rys Farthing identify some important criteria for distinguishing 'good' research, particularly highlighting the key role of the values and ethics of practitioner-researchers. In acknowledging the potentially fraught relationship between research, policy and practice, Farthing and Bessant explore the wider political context in which this is set. This includes the identification of methods, processes and tactics that are involved in successfully engaging and communicating research findings to a range of differing key audiences. The chapter encourages practitioner-researchers to be alert to structures and relations of power, politics and the 'truth claims' that they might make for their work, arguing that these matters have crucial significance in the way that particular messages are heard and understood by the audiences and consumers of research findings.

Finally, Chapter 10 explores the broad policy and practice context within which research *with* young people and on services *for* young people is undertaken. Drawing on work by Silverman and Bloor, Cullen and Bradford identify potential positions or roles that might be adopted by social researchers, and relate these to the work of practitioner-researchers. The chapter goes on to take a critical view of so-called evidence-based policy and practice, and concludes by exploring the contribution that the practitioner-researcher might make to policy and practice in contemporary work with young people.

# 1 Working as a practitioner-researcher

Fin Cullen, Simon Bradford and Laura Green

## Overview

This collection is aimed at practitioner-researchers working within the field of young people's services. If you are reading this book, you are perhaps completing a dissertation as part of a university course. You may be a practitioner or manager attempting to develop a research-led approach to policy and practice at your organisation. This chapter explores the nature of practitioner research, and outlines some of the possible tensions and conflicts that can arise when entering the field while acting as practitioner *and* researcher simultaneously. It explores and outlines various notions of participatory action research and praxis, in relation to how research-orientated approaches can directly influence and shape policy and practice.

Our key questions include:

- What is research for?
- What is your role as practitioner-researcher when conducting your study?

The research in which you are involved may be about developing and evaluating local services, producing a needs assessment or community profile, or activating change for a practice-based problem. However, your research may have a more theoretical basis, or may be about creating new knowledge in other fields. With this in mind, it is essential that you are clear about your study's focus, purpose and audience. The research-based work evaluation for funders or management will be substantially different in tone and focus, for example, from an academic dissertation. For instance, the role of research may be a key part of the descriptors used to map your professional role. Currently, the UK National Occupational Standards for youth work stress the need for youth workers to be aware of the tools and processes involved in evaluating day-to-day youth work practice including involving young people in the evaluation process.[1]

The following chapters aim to highlight the main debates in the area, in addition to guiding practitioners towards further materials that can develop research skills and support their work as practitioner-researchers. Given that the UK National Occupational

Standards' practitioner-oriented definition of youth work incorporates a research and evaluation element, it might seem that participatory and action research approaches have a key role in developing both research and youth work practice. Increasingly, many youth practitioners are expected to take larger roles in planning and evaluating practice interventions, in addition to evidencing youth work via a range of qualitative approaches to data collection and the accumulation of quantitative indicators.

The kinds of research you may have in mind may vary considerably – from small-scale consultations looking at young people's needs in a small geographical area, to larger community profiles or evaluations of youth services and education programmes, to theoretically driven work that could form a Master's dissertation. This chapter aims to encourage readers to think critically about what it means to be a practitioner *and* a researcher, and how those identities may complement or clash with each other. We will consider how you might think critically about the nature of power and ethics, how the research agenda is shaped and to what ends. Whilst being a practitioner-researcher might enable you to reflect critically on your practice, improve service delivery and make key links between theory, policy and practice, it may also pose significant challenges about what and whom research is for, and where your role as a researcher begins and ends.

In defining social research and practitioner research, in particular, we borrow from Barrett *et al.* (1999), and argue that research in education and the social sciences is always characterised by at least five principles. Your research should be *systematic*, *critical* and *self-critical enquiry* that aims to contribute to advancing *knowledge* and/or *practice*. In thinking through and planning your own research you should consider the extent to which you are able to meet these basic criteria for good research.

We refer to each element briefly in turn.

## Systematic

By this, we mean that research should be conducted in a way that is planned; it should be completed in an appropriate sequence; and it should have a clear rationale. Anyone reading your work should be able to understand exactly how you went about the research and the reasons why you did it in that way. When you write up your work (in either a dissertation or a research paper), your writing should reflect the rationale that underlies the work itself.

## Critical

In social research, criticality and the adoption of a critical stance are fundamental. This means that you should scrutinise everything that you do, everything that you are told and all that you infer from your completed research. It means continually asking *how* and *why* questions ('How can I best research that question?', 'Why should I do it this way?', and so on). You should also adopt this stance in relation to your reading: look for the possible reasons *why* some claim that a writer makes might not be true or correct. *How* is the writer making her arguments and to what extent does that represent a *particular* position rather than a general truth, as claimed? Criticality will help you to become more sensitive to the nature of argument and truth claims.

## Self-critical

Being self-critical takes the idea of criticality a little further and helps you to focus on you the researcher. Being self-critical means that we have to think about our own *position* in the research and as a researcher (sometimes referred to as *positionality*). We have to be very clear about who we are as researchers and what we bring with us. For example, the fact that I am a white middle-aged man or a black woman from a certain class background may mean that I have particular ways of understanding the world around me. How might that understanding shape the way I choose particular research questions and go about researching them? How might it encourage me to understand the responses made by participants? What impact does my identity or my values have on interpreting the significance of those responses? Being self-critical applies to every aspect of social research, from the beginning of the project to its conclusion.

## Enquiry

Social research probably starts with a sense of curiosity and an interest in a particular question or puzzle that emerges in your practice or more broadly in your professional or academic life. It might simply be concerned with asking the question 'What's going on here?' or it may be something much more complex about aspects of policy, organisation, management, young people's lives and experience, and so on. This means that in planning your research project you should have an explicit purpose in mind.

## Knowledge and practice

We argue that your research project (i.e. what your research is for) should make a contribution to knowledge about young people, communities or services for young people and communities (depending on your research question). Because you are a practitioner-researcher, it should also contribute to the development of practice, where possible. Your work should therefore make a contribution to what we know and what we can do.

All social research studies need a clearly identifiable research question as a starting point. This question establishes the boundaries of the enquiry, the parameters of the study, and enables researchers to develop and design a clear research strategy – including methodological and epistemological framing. The kinds of theory underpinning researchers' understanding of the social world often pose different kinds of research question, and such differing questions need different methods. For example, if a researcher were interested in measuring levels of homophobic bullying, a question such as the following might be posed:

- What were the levels of reported homophobic bullying incidents in secondary schools in the last year?

This research question concerns the social problem of 'homophobic bullying' and seeks to establish the level of this problem in schools. The question suggests using a largely quantitative approach. This might include statistical analysis of reported incidents and questionnaires for institutions, and also involve reviewing school homophobic and general bullying policies, and the reporting protocols that are in place. This would provide empirical measures that could be used across time and location to identify whether levels of bullying had changed, and whether this was an issue in particular school locations, or amongst particular groups of students.

A researcher who is interested in lesbian, gay and bisexual young people's personal experiences of the social world might pose a different question, such as:

- How do young gay, lesbian and bisexual people narrate their experience of 'coming out' in school?

This question is about trying to grasp the ways in which these young people's accounts provide understanding of individual pupils' experiences of being 'out' in educational spaces. The question suggests a plan that incorporates such methods as individual and/or group interviews rather than large-scale questionnaires, in order to capture individual and group narratives. Whilst such a study could not provide the comparative statistics offered by the previous homophobic bullying question, narratives of bullying as a lived experience may be present in the students' accounts. Similarly, LGB students may also have accounts that do not involve bullying, and may instead include positive experiences and acceptance in school. Of course, a researcher may choose to take a blended, multi-method approach, combining both quantitative and qualitative methods.

The point here is that particular epistemological framings and research aims shape the kinds of question and methods used. Whilst both research questions are interested in sexualities and schooling, and the findings may touch on the 'social problem' of homophobic bullying, each would have a distinct set of methods shaped by the different macro and micro understandings and perspectives of knowledge in the school settings. Both research questions would also be potentially insightful in creating policy and practice interventions within educational settings.

*Epistemology* is a term used to describe the theory of knowledge: how do we know what we think we know? There have been a number of main traditions that sociologists have used to frame their particular approaches epistemologically to social research. We will briefly consider two here: positivism and interpretivism.

*Positivism* arose at the inception of many of the social science disciplines. At its heart is the notion that researchers can study society in a scientific way. There have been various proponents of positivist methods throughout the history of sociology, including such notable, and very different, sociologists as Emile Durkheim and Talcott Parsons. Positivism adopted many methods directly from the natural sciences, and has an emphasis on collecting what Durkheim referred to as 'social facts'. By analysing such 'facts', sociologists are believed to be able to provide scientific explanations for social events, and identify solutions for social problems in order to develop and shape theories about society.

The second influential approach, *interpretivism*, is often associated with such sociologists as Max Weber and Georg Simmel. This places the emphasis not on the collection of *social facts*, but rather on understanding the accounts and the meaning making and social significance people have about their social worlds. Such an approach highlights multiple 'realities', in opposition to the Durkheimian position that emphasises that 'social facts' (broadly speaking, culture and 'collective representations': all the shared meanings, symbols and ways in which we understand who we are) are external to and constraining of individual conduct. Such sociological traditions frame the nature of critical enquiry and understandings, and these approaches shape the research methods, mode of analysis and claims one might make for data.

## What is practitioner research?

Our broad argument is that research, as an activity, constitutes a vital and rich space where youth practitioners may engage critically with debates from the field, policy and practice, and link theory and practice. In and of itself, research provides scope for self-reflection, and personal and practitioner development, beyond that the development of knowledge for its own sake, or an examination of how one might develop progressive practice in any given area.

Everyday practice for many contemporary youth practitioners will include various forms of data gathering, recordings, needs assessments, and programme and project evaluations. The push for 'evidence' in many youth settings may sometimes seem to be activated on the basis of particular empirical measures – those of accredited and recorded outcomes, school league tables, about demographic, descriptive user statistics, and quick-run surveys. However, Issitt and Spence (2005: 63) note: 'face to face practice, by its very nature is not concerned primarily with gathering evidence and creating meaning, but rather with personal and social change'. The kinds of change perceived as important by face-to-face practitioners may be of little interest or legibility in the kinds of evidence criteria and empirical measures required by policy and practice settings. Such differences in recognising and perceiving change between practitioners and policy-makers/funders might suggest that a broader base of empirical measures and 'evidence' may be necessary in order to capture this wider range of activity and meaning in practice settings.

Whilst data gathering as an exercise may be an everyday part of youth practice, this differs significantly from social research, in that the latter is orientated around an inquiry to provide deeper understandings of the social world and/or in response to a sociological problem. The kinds of 'evidence' and data that practitioners are asked to gather, and that might be seen as persuasive in securing further funding or justifying the existence of a youth project, are often largely quantitative (i.e. numerical and statistical data) in order to be included in wider metric measures. For example, in recent years, UK youth services have often produced Best Value Performance Indicators to demonstrate the cost effectiveness and reach of local services in relation to percentages of local young people participating in local youth activities and/or achieving accreditation. Youth practitioners may collect data of that kind for their youth project, yet this form of ongoing monitoring differs from social research in the kinds of knowledge produced. The data gathering is primarily based on attempting to demonstrate outcomes through cost effectiveness and achievement of pre-defined policy aims, for example, rather than on solving sociological problems or providing theoretical analysis of the cultural and material practices of youth services and young people's participation.

Thus, one of the key questions any practitioner needs to consider is whether, for instance, 'good youth practice' is in any way the same as 'good research'. For example, the UK based National Youth Agency currently defines youth work as:

> Youth work helps young people learn about themselves, others and society, through informal educational activities which combine enjoyment, challenge and learning . . . [Youth workers seek] to promote young people's personal and social development and enable them to have a voice, influence and place in their communities and society as a whole.[2]

McLeod (1999: 8) defines practitioner research as 'research carried out by practitioners for the purpose of advancing their own practice'. This somewhat limited definition orientates practitioner to research in the realm of personal practice – perhaps in developing or evaluating interventions, or possibly in advancing the skill base of the practitioner. However, McLeod's definition has been seen as somewhat simplistic and reductive; after all, practitioner research is often concerned with a much broader realm beyond that of personal development and practice (Shaw 2005).

Indeed, Shaw (2005: 1231–1232) suggests a more critical engagement with the relationship between 'mainstream' academic and practitioner research and asks:

> What is the relationship between practitioner research and 'mainstream' academic social work research? Is practitioner research simply a street market version of mainstream research, or is it a distinctive genre of research? What is the quality and value of such research?

Whilst Shaw is examining social work, the questions about the interface between academic research and practice are deeply pertinent. Shaw's argument is that much practitioner research has been perceived as 'employer-led, "applied", and based on an expectation that it should lead to results that are directly useful' (Shaw 2005: 1242). We concur that practitioner research has both the capacity and the capability to be rigorous and critically engaged with debates within policy and theory. We would also contest limitations or lower expectations of practitioner research as being fundamentally a separate genre of research from 'mainstream' forms, or an intellectually diminished version of academic work. Indeed, these approaches are not necessarily exclusive. One might simultaneously move towards a progressive practice, generate new social theory *and* provide a forum for critical reflection as a practitioner.

We also maintain that there is a range of ways that practitioner-based research should be acknowledged as having particular value. We identify four here:

1 Generating insights from a practitioner perspective in order to improve and develop practice.
2 The capacity for research-informed critically reflective practice to activate broad social change.
3 Using a practice base to generate theory and influence policy.
4 As an important stage of staff development in its capacity to provide spaces for critical reflection.

This is broadly what we discussed earlier in arguing that research should contribute to the production of new knowledge that can advance practice (i.e. develop or improve practice). We also think that the generation of knowledge to develop theory (i.e. knowledge that can develop our understanding of the social world and improve our explanations of how it changes, develops or remains the same) is a crucial responsibility for social researchers generally, and for practitioner-researchers specifically. However, to do that means a strategic and responsive approach that moves beyond the kinds of 'evidence' that you may be collecting as part of your everyday practice, and towards some of the approaches detailed in this volume. Your research may involve collaborative work with colleagues and young people for one or more of the objectives referred to above.

## Who are the practitioner-researchers?

Scholars have identified practitioner research as a growing area within health, education, welfare and youth services (Jarvis 1999; McLeod 1999; McWilliam 2004; Shaw 2005; Sikes and Potts 2008; West 1999). Indeed, Sikes and Potts (2008) note that there are growing numbers of 'insider' researchers studying within education, health and welfare organisations, through either their continuing professional higher education or the mainstreaming of research as an active part of professional development within many practice settings. Scholars acknowledge the heterogeneity of both practice and research in the wide range of practitioner-researcher settings, and the varying motivations of this diverse group (Jarvis 1999; Sikes and Potts 2008). Practitioner-researchers thus include undergraduate and postgraduate students, those in employment settings tasked to develop small projects to influence policy decisions, others involved in internal team evaluations, and 'others who undertake research to satisfy their own curiosity. These are practitioner-researchers, but they are often not recognised as researchers' (Jarvis 1999: 7).

Jarvis's (1999) description of practitioner-researchers highlights the issue that practitioners who undertake research may be not be recognised by their 'research' endeavours. Pertinent issues here include those of authenticity and 'expert' knowledge in the realms of both youth practice *and* social research. It is important that practitioner-researchers clearly identify how they will navigate the twin issues of recognition and expertise in developing and disseminating their research.

However, there remains tension. Research, as an activity, might be perceived as the preserve of research 'experts', and 'expert practitioners' may struggle to identify themselves within this dual role. The expertise here springs largely from the kinds of reified knowledge that 'expert' researchers may seem to possess about epistemology (the theory of knowledge), methodology and ethics, and how this might translate or be engaged with in the realm of the practitioner.

This is particularly important when practitioner-researchers are involved in exploring their home organisation and area of practice, perhaps even focusing on their work with colleagues and clients in a particular youth setting. Within such fields as youth work, notions of 'expertise' may also be contentious, inasmuch as what it means to be a youth practitioner, a professional and an expert researcher might be contested both within and outside the field. However, we would also argue that 'expert' research knowledge is an important area to be acquired if practitioner research is to be effective in building new knowledge in the arenas of theory, policy and practice.

## What is distinctive about practitioner research?

There is a wide variety of purpose, focus and methods used within practitioner research. Not all practitioner-researchers conduct research that has a direct applied focus on practice; nor do they necessarily conduct research in their own practice context. Importantly, then, when assuming the identity of practitioner-researcher, one should remain *critical*. As a researcher and a practitioner you need to be mindful of the overarching purpose of the research, the processes of knowledge production, and the kinds of knowledge and evidence that may be produced in a particular context. In order to explore the possible range and scope of practitioner research within youth work and other allied fields, it is important to consider the purposes of social research more broadly, both within and outside university and other research institutes. It is helpful to consider the status and claims of different kinds of knowledge in policy and practice settings. Bloor (1997) highlights the criticism that has developed around the focus and nature of knowledge in debates over the purpose and use of social research in directly influencing policy and practice. Critics of practitioner research point to the 'unscientific' nature of unqualified researchers conducting social enquiry, and questions are raised over whether practitioner knowledge is the same as scientific knowledge.

> The other strand of criticism of practice-orientated social research is that articulated by commentators such as Schön (1983), who have followed Schutz (1962) in arguing that professional work does not entail the deployment of scientific knowledge, but rather involves the deployment of a different kind of knowledge altogether, knowledge-in-action, which is rigorous but not comprehensive, task-orientated but not systematic, and experiential rather than research based. In this reading, social research has little of value to contribute to practitioners' work.
>
> (Bloor 1997: 223)

However, as Bloor later notes, if the research is directly interested in considering practitioners' everyday work as its topic, then it does require the systematic research-based deployment of scientific knowledge, which is thus not necessarily constructed as separate and distinct from the realm of knowledge-in-practice.

Some of these debates that attempt to locate the 'right' types of objective and 'scientific knowledge' replicate those within feminist research. In such areas, experiential and subjective knowledge may be perceived to be sufficiently lacking in systematic rigour, in comparison to the earlier traditions within the social sciences of large-scale studies searching for social 'facts'. Feminist critiques have framed the need to challenge androcentric and elitist constructions of scientific knowledge (Stanley and Wise 1993). Whilst such a critique seems to posit 'scientific knowledge' as almost an omnipotent, large-scale kind of knowing, the small-scale, detailed focus of other kinds of practice-based knowledge is seemingly diminished. We argue that both traditions are valuable in different settings and in relation to particular research problems. There are established and valuable traditions within qualitative social science research that are specifically orientated to small-scale, rich analysis of people's social worlds – the interpretivist tradition (what Geertz (1973) calls 'thick description') that we mentioned earlier. Practitioner-orientated research, which often takes small-scale and qualitative approaches, enables practitioners and researchers to develop a deeper relationship with the field and focus on everyday practice. Bloor (1997) argues that this focus will encourage practitioners to engage further with such debates in social research.

Others critics of practitioner research doubt the transferability and representativeness of 'small scale "me-focused" studies' and view the apparently theory-free orientation of practice enquiry as a kind of 'flabby new humanism' (McWilliam 2004: 114). Yet, as we highlight throughout this volume, practitioner research does not always take a qualitative approach; nor is it necessarily always primarily interested in directly influencing practice. However, practitioner research can and often does engage deeply with theory, and can take a variety of forms, from small-scale insider studies to larger-scale comparative quantitative enquiry, and such a range of methodological perspectives frames the chapters within this volume.

Before we go on to explore approaches used by practitioner-researchers in the field, it is worthwhile considering what we think is the distinctiveness of practitioner knowledge. McWilliam (2004) notes that advocates of practitioner research make many claims, including that such *insider* work is somehow 'more authentic' and 'more ethical' than traditional forms of *outsider* research. Explicit within this notion is that 'practitioner research has more potential to give voice to the voiceless, amplifying rather than submerging marginal populations and projects' (McWilliam 2004: 114). This emphasis on the experiential is in itself a central part of modern youth work traditions and modes of informal learning. However, despite claims for 'authenticity', one might wish to trouble such claims and call for a more nuanced approach that critically interrogates both the nature of practice and the kinds of knowledge held by the practitioner research community.

The notion of 'reflexivity' – widely used within social research – is useful here in adopting the critical and self-critical stance we highlighted earlier. Many practitioners may already be familiar with ideas of critical reflection within practice settings, in both challenging and exploring practice as a technical exercise and reflecting on the practitioner's role and the broader structural approaches to practice. A tradition of reflexivity lies within social science research. Reflexivity concerns an awareness that the researcher cannot be detached and stand outside the subject matter when conducting social research. This may also incorporate social researchers' exploring personal reflections on their values, politics, social status, relationships and experiences and how these shape and influence their research.

If we accept that social research is not a value-free exercise, then the notion of research reflexivity enables the social researcher to think critically about the nature of the research, the claims made for the data, the positionality of the researcher, and the ethical framing of the research. Such reflexivity within practitioner research would focus on the research process, relationships, and the claims made for the data, and would critically reflect on claims of 'authenticity' and the process of knowledge production.

This is not to say that practitioner-orientated work cannot be highly illuminating (and reflexive) in exploring tensions between theory, policy and practice. Too often, practitioner knowledge might be seen as mainly linear and primarily orientated towards securing change in practice. This is a worthwhile and useful tradition, but we would argue that practitioner-based research also has the capacity to provide robust dialogues and the generation of new theoretical frames that may speak to existing theory and policy.

## Practice-based task 1.1 The practitioner-researcher role

Consider the following:

- First, create a list of your current work activities in your present role as a youth practitioner.
- Create a list of the activities you will be involved with as a social researcher.
- How much of an overlap is there between these two roles? For example, will your research take place in the same physical spaces with the same client group during your youth practice?
- Discuss with a fellow student or in your research journal how you might manage the different emphasis and agenda in these roles.
- Finally, take some time to design information and guidance sheets to explain your research idea for use with young participants and their parents/carers. This should be designed in line with the capacity and age group of your imagined participants.

## Action research and participatory approaches

The previous section highlighted practitioner research's many forms and purposes. This section explores one approach that has been linked to practitioner research for over three decades, and more recently orientated towards the 'what works' agenda: *action research*. The purpose is to introduce action research and explore a range of action research-related approaches that have previously been utilised in education and community work settings by practitioner-researchers. This will include various forms of action research and participatory action research. We discuss action research here as part of a wider framework that may be of potential use for those attempting to combine youth work and/or educational practice and research. Indeed, many of the following chapters discuss research methods that may be used alone or in combination within or outside a wider action research project. Action research provides a focus here, as it is a broad approach that can be amenable to practice-orientated contexts, especially when practitioners wish to initiate change and critically reflect on practice.

Various definitions of action research are commonly used in academic and practice contexts. However, the 'action' aspect revolves around practicality, with action researchers enabling a change within a practice context. As Frisby, Maguire and Reid (2009: 14) write: 'Action research aims to bring theory, method, and practice as people work collaboratively towards practical outcomes and new forms of understanding.' This linking of theory and practice and the power mechanisms in play in particular settings enables practitioners to use action research as a site of critical self-reflection. As Carr and Kemmis (1986: 162) note: 'Action research is simply a form of self-reflective enquiry undertaken by participants in social situations in order to improve the rationality and justice of their own practices, their understanding of these practices, and the situations in which the practices are carried out.'

A highly flexible, dynamic action research approach can use a combination of quantitative and qualitative methods, and thus may incorporate survey data, focus groups, participant observations, and practitioner reflection. Action research has thus proved highly popular amongst practitioners seeking to initiate change or seek solutions to practice-orientated issues. Over the past four decades, action research has also been particularly influential in education and youth practitioner-based contexts, as it owes much to 'ground up' solutions and has a capacity to be participatory in involving other practitioners and young people. As Rapoport (1970: 499) states: 'Action research is a type of applied social research differing from other varieties in the immediacy of the researcher's involvement in the action process.'

Action research has been used in several different ways. Rapoport (1970) perceives researchers as 'change agents' (Bennis 1966) seeking solutions through joint collaboration, and certainly one might thus see its clear use in community work and other educational settings. Kurt Lewin's (1948) spiral cycle of *planning–acting–observing–reflecting* may be familiar to many readers who already use a similar model of experiential learning within their everyday youth work or education practice. Lewin's model is based on the idea of action research being a form of democratic practice, and as such it has been highly influential in education research with its emphasis on the values of the practitioner (Robson 1993). Such applications mean that models of action research have been especially prevalent in such areas as education, community development and youth work research traditions.

We suggest that the various approaches and methods that constitute action research have particular relevance to the work of youth practitioners especially, because the methodology has a focus on experience, and participation has much relevance to the kinds of enquiry and the values inherent in the everyday work undertaken within the field. Moreover, within some of the earlier traditions, commitment to 'praxis' (a kind of theoretically informed practice) reflects the value base of many working within informal education and youth settings in linking and developing theory into a committed practice that might be seen to shape the everyday world (Smith 1999: 1).

*Participatory action research* (PAR) takes these ideas some steps further in developing a commitment to working collaboratively with the 'researched'. Many readers will be familiar with the participatory practices that form an everyday part of their work, and are enshrined within (at least the rhetoric of) public service policy. Of course, the levels and capacity for such 'youth participation' vary from organisation to organisation and within projects that actively seek young people to become active as researchers and participants.

Research *with* and *by* young people has had growing significance in recent years in academic, policy and practice arenas. For many youth workers reading this chapter, empowerment-based approaches stressing self-advocacy and the political engagement of young people will be far from new. Of course, practitioners may experience limits in how they might develop emancipatory research practice in youth work and education settings when faced with the conflicting challenges and tensions of everyday practice demands. As a youth practitioner, you may work collaboratively with young people as co-researchers to examine a given collaboratively defined research problem. Such an approach emphasises aspects of process and has a 'commitment to research contribution and "giving back" to community collaborators' (Cahill 2007: 298). Such an emphasis on process, participation and social justice remains at the heart of the mainstream traditions of much youth work practice (West 1999). Again, PAR may thus represent a 'good fit' for many practitioners, with the approaches and methods widely used within such arenas as youth work, informal education and community development. Indeed, Cahill (2007) argues that PAR offers a helpful framework for community practitioners working towards social justice and democratising the research process, particularly when working with relatively disempowered groups, such as young people. In such participatory approaches both young people and youth practitioners would work collaboratively as agents of change in the research process.

However, there are key differences between everyday youth practice and sites of critical enquiry. Whether your role is as a youth worker, educator or youth justice worker, the main thrust of your everyday practice is usually not about systematically generating new knowledge and theorising about social worlds, beyond that of youth practice orientation. The various action research models have not been without their critics.

From a traditional social science perspective, action research approaches may be seen as lacking rigour, and from a positivist stance, they have been criticised for failing to achieve the necessary detached 'objectivity'. Within academic and practice contexts it may not be feasible for young people to be involved in all stages of the research process, including the initial research design, especially when acknowledging funding deadlines or the requirements of an academic course. Indeed, young people may not be interested in or familiar with some of the abstract theoretical analysis that sometimes characterises academically orientated research. Yet this does not suggest that participatory approaches should be deployed only in applied and/or practice contexts. Cahill's work connects with theoretical work considering the construction of knowledge and the purpose and nature of education and research (Cahill 2004, 2007).

### Case study 1.1
### A feminist participatory action research project

As a practitioner-researcher, Laura undertook Ph.D. research within girls-only youth and community work settings. The project investigated possibilities for flexible sports participation with non-active girls. The research project used feminist participatory action research (FPAR). FPAR is participatory; defined by the need for action; and creates knowledge, but not for the sake of knowledge alone. By using FPAR within youth and community settings, two groups of young women (a young mums' group and a young women's group) were encouraged to examine their experiences and develop sports projects that suited their diverse needs and values. Research proceeded through three broad phases:

1 Interactive group discussion activities opened up debates about contradictory discourses of femininity and sport, exposed fears and concerns, and began to unpick patterns of disengagement.
2 Planning of needs-led physical activity projects. Youth groups were given full responsibility to select sports/physical activities, and where, how and when they wanted to participate. Young women collaboratively debated which activities they felt able to participate in and which they wished to avoid, and applied for project funding. They recruited, interviewed and employed female coaches.
3 Participating in and evaluating the projects.

The highlight of the project was the movement of initially 'non-sporty' young women into eventually engaging in and enjoying physical activity. Initially, young women often voiced negative opinions towards sport, but by the completion they evaluated their experiences as enjoyable and exciting. Both young women's groups participated in further youth-led physical activity projects following the completion of the research.

There were a number of key challenges facing this research approach, particularly around the differing expectations of all of the project stakeholders (young women, funders, university regulators, and local authority managers), whilst at the same time ensuring the collection of useful data. The priorities of other stakeholders conflicted with the priorities of the young women and the research goals: for example, funders contributed financial backing but subsequently specified activities on which this could be spent, which limited the young women's autonomy on the project. The practitioner-researcher identified a range of ways to aid balancing these conflicting demands via the use of service-level agreements and developing an ongoing dialogue between stake-holders.

Another significant challenge was the need to distinguish between 'good research' and 'good youth work'. This balance needed constant attention throughout the projects: for example, in balancing a participatory structure in which the young women led the projects against risks of overburdening or creating a feeling of obligation, and acknowledging that young people were not inclined to participate in all aspects of the research process (data analysis).

Collaborative approaches create space for young people to be creative, reflective and innovative, and to develop projects that meet their own diverse needs and desires and from which they can learn much. Youth work settings are often ideal sites for carrying out such research approaches, as the core values and emphasis on relationship building of youth work and FPAR mesh together extremely well. Youth work practitioner-researchers are ideally placed to deliver these kinds of projects by drawing on their professional skills and credibility both within organisations and with young people. The FPAR approach in this case study created an environment of mutual, informal learning with an emphasis on possibilities for reciprocity between researcher and participants. However, this was not always a smooth process and FPAR facilitators must be mindful of potentially challenging ethical issues that arise within the research/practice context.

---

There remain potential limits and challenges to the suitability and scope of participatory approaches such as PAR and FPAR in some practice contexts, especially when working in highly sensitive or specialist areas. In an exploration of how youth participation agendas were taken up on the ground in UK-based children and young people's services, Middleton (2006) found that such opportunities remained patchy; and where youth participation existed, these approaches remained of limited popularity with young people. This resulted in a fairly limited group of self-selecting young people becoming actively involved, thus limiting project claims about representativeness.

PAR approaches within youth work and education contexts are often framed within peer *education* and enquiry. Many practitioners will be familiar with the idea of 'peer education'. However, the notion of 'peer' is itself fraught with difficulties. Young people may have very little in common, other than chronological age, with other 'youth'; and whilst generational separation may emerge because of policy contexts and practice delivery settings, young people may not be able to provide insights with other young people simply because they are all aged sixteen. Wider structural issues, such as gender, ethnicity, culture and social class, come to have a place in creating the capacity and space for such research interactions and engagement. As critiques of peer education approaches have been careful to point out (Bessant 2003; Bragg 2007), these might be perceived as a kind of 'ventriloquism', where young people are set up as 'experts' in educating or researching their peers for what remains an 'adult' policy-driven agenda in which notions of 'authenticity' and voice need to be opened up to critique. As Heath *et al.* (2009: 70) argue: 'There is a danger that where a specially selected group of young people are actively involved in research it will be assumed that this research is therefore a more valid representation of the views and experiences of all young people.'

The difficulties and challenges around tokenistic involvement might be overcome by focusing on topics that have a direct relevance to young people. This particularly under-lines much of the participatory research work supported by the UK National Youth Agency but remains problematic for those researchers who may want to explore more theoretical and/or abstract concerns. Similarly, unequal power relations are not fully negated through the use of peer and participatory research approaches, although many advocates for participatory youth research have taken a variety of approaches to diminish such inequalities. Readers already familiar with the much-used Hart's ladder (Hart 1992) will acknowledge the limits of such a model. 'Poor' participatory approaches may leave research with and by young people at the lower rungs of manipulation, decoration and tokenism (Cahill 2007). However, although versions of this ladder have been drawn

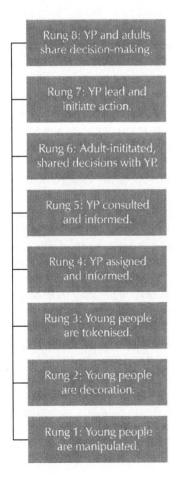

**Figure 1.1** Hart's ladder of youth participation

*Note:* Hart identifies Rungs 1–3 as forms of non-participation

*Source:* Hart (1992)

on in citizen involvement, user participation and volunteer action approaches, there remain some severe limitations with this model. For example, the metaphor of a ladder imagines a gauged level of involvement and does not completely engage with an individual or groups' starting point or capacity for engagement.

## Ethics, power and practice: what is research ethics?

Social research in common with youth practice is not a value-free exercise, but is deeply enmeshed in the power dynamics of the wider social world and the politics in play within these research settings. As a practitioner-researcher your research *and* youth practice are thus fundamentally shaped by power relations, especially in terms of your capacity to identify the area of research and consider who might be seen as the research subject. This holds true whether you choose to conduct research on home territory (your youth club, project, tutor group, etc.) or move into other spaces – for example, in the wider assessment of community projects in a neighbourhood.

A range of definitions of 'ethics' focuses on notions of appropriate behaviour around the 'morality of human conduct' (Edwards and Mauthner 2002: 14). Ethical principles within social research are usually focused on consent, privacy, respect, deception, harm and confidentiality. Readers can find details of how to find a range of national social research organisational codes at the end of this chapter. Later, Rogers and Ludhra in Chapter 3 consider the issue of research ethics in greater detail. At this point, we briefly want to touch on issues of practice and research ethics and values. The power dynamics within social research in youth settings are multiple and complex. As Case study 1.1 highlights, even in a setting that may appear conducive to participatory and youth-led approaches, there remain key challenges deriving from power disparities. Focusing on youth work, West (1999: 183) writes: 'the relations of power are threefold: first, power of the adult (youth worker) over young people; second, power of the researcher over the researched; and third, power of professional over client group'. This means that the power relations within a research project must be critically examined, and participants should be protected from undue harm and distress resulting from involvement in the study. Practitioner research conjures up specific ethical dilemmas in the workplace, in which relationships can be significantly changed (Sikes and Potts 2008). Not all youth practitioner-researchers may focus on the experiences of youth; indeed, you may be evaluating services and/or the experiences of other professionals. This may include the kinds of scrutinising and audit practices that have emerged within inspection regimes, such as Ofsted in the UK. To these we can add the growing use of peer review and observation within practice settings, which can lead to professionals feeling that they are under the researcher's gaze (Perryman 2006; Sikes and Potts 2008).

These substantive issues of power in *who* establishes the research agenda, analyses the data and writes up and disseminates the research, and for what purpose, can fundamentally impact on peer relations within a practice setting. Ethical issues within intra and inter-professional research might include the real dynamics and possibilities of whistle blowing or substantially altering workplace relations beyond that of the study (Sikes and Potts 2008).

Moreover, ethical dilemmas are also present in the changing focus and dimensions entailed in youth practitioners altering their relationships with young people to become researchers with young people within their overall professional capacity. Key to this is reflecting on how you might manage research and practice relations before, during and after fieldwork, in order to cause no harm to other colleagues, clients or indeed yourself as a practitioner-researcher (Sikes and Potts 2008).

## Practice-based task 1.2  Research ethics

Either in a research journal or with a colleague, discuss the following:

- What policies and procedures, such as confidentiality, child protection and information-sharing protocols, are you obliged to uphold as a practitioner in your current work setting?
- How might these policies impact on the scope for research with either young people or fellow practitioners in your work setting?

There is a need here to be mindful of the significant ethical dimensions of entering the field in the dual role of researcher *and* practitioner. As a practitioner, you are probably familiar with the various codes of ethics, licensing procedures and ethical guidance from various professional associations. If you are a youth worker, your work will be guided by codes of professional practice, such as those published by the UK National Youth Agency, as well as local agency guidance on confidentiality and child protection. Such guidance often outlines the kinds of 'professional' behaviour, boundaries, and structures of accountability that organise your practice. On the other hand, you will probably also be required to follow institutional ethical codes for social researchers.

Such dual guidance positions (professional and research) may sometimes conflict, so planning and design issues, such as child protection and the limits of confidentiality and 'informed consent', need to be carefully thought through before commencing the research. At the end of this chapter there are web addresses for obtaining research ethics guidance that can provide an initial foundation to how practitioners manage these potentially competing and conflicting codes. When working as a practitioner-researcher, the specifically *ethical* dimension of research practice may go beyond the requirements that may be covered in a professional code of practice. When one is working as a researcher, particularly within one's home organisation and with a regular client group, questions of power, consent and coercion become especially salient.

Youth professionals regularly navigate the tensions and clashing priorities of professionalism *and* professional values and organisational demands (McCulloch 2009). Ethical practice is thus contextual, situational and relational, negotiated in line with the prevailing situation and the obligations and tensions of any given setting. Whilst 'participatory' approaches may at first glance appear more clearly aligned with national statements of the values within many youth and educational practices than traditional forms of 'outsider' research, the kinds of knowledge production undertaken, the setting and the context, all impact on how a practitioner-researcher may negotiate a contextual ethical practice. Working out what counts as ethical research practice means taking all of these into account. These ideas are developed further throughout this volume.

## Summary of main points

In summary, the main issues we have explored so far are:

- Your research should aim to be a systematic, critical and self-critical enquiry to create new knowledge.
- Practitioner research may be done for a variety of reasons to shape theory, policy and practice.
- Many scholars have attempted to make special claims for the value of practitioner research.
- Practitioner-researchers need to reflect critically on their 'insider' role and the ethical and power issues this may have on their research.
- Action research and participatory approaches are used within practitioner research in social work, education, community and youth work.

## Further reading

For an overview of the role of practitioner-researchers, Jarvis (1999) is a good starting point.

Jarvis, P. (1999) *The Practitioner-Researcher: Developing theory from practice*, New York: John Wiley and Sons.

If you decide to take a participatory approach, there are a number of useful introductory resources in the area. Kellet (2005) takes a step-by-step approach to explain how to support children within a school setting in research design, collection and analysis. Kirby (1999) provides an overview of ethical and procedural issues when involving young people in research projects. The more recent collection by Tisdall *et al.* (2009) provides a range of case studies and practical examples of activities for potential researchers to explore the range of questions arising before entering the field.

Kellett, M. (2005) *How to Develop Children as Researchers: A step-by-step guide to the research process*, London: Sage.
Kirby, P. (1999) *Involving Young Researchers*, York: York Publishing Services.
Tisdall, E., Davis, J.M. and Gallagher, M. (2009) *Research with Children and Young People: Research design, methods and analysis*, London: Sage.

## Research ethics resources

Many researchers follow the ethical procedures in place at their home institutions, for example, by submitting an application to the university research ethics committee. Various national and international research organisations produce guidance on ethical research for social researchers. In addition, some NGOs, such as Barnardo's, publish particular codes of ethics for their social researchers working with children and young people.

- The British Educational Research Association website: http://www.bera.ac.uk/publications/guides.php._
- National Youth Agency (UK) website: http://nya.org.uk/dynamic_files/yrn/toolkit/Stage%206%20YRN%20Toolkit.pdf.

Ethical codes for youth workers can be found in:

- National Youth Agency (1999) *Ethics in Youth Work*, Leicester: NYA.
- Youth Action and Policy Association, NSW (Australia) website: http://www.yapa.org.au/youthwork/ethics/codetextwithcomment.php.

## Notes

1   Find a full list of National Occupational Standards for Youth and Community Work at: http://www.lluk.org/wp-content/uploads/2010/11/National-Occupational-Standards-for-Youth-Work.pdf.
2   See http://www.nya.org.uk.

## References

Barrett, E., Lally, V., Thresh, R. and Purcell, S. (1999) *Signposts for Educational Research*, London: Sage.

Bennis, W. (1966) *Changing Organizations: Essays on the development and evolution of human organization*, New York: McGraw-Hill.

Bessant, J. (2003) 'Youth participation, a new mode of government', *Policy Studies*, 24 (2/3): 87–100.

Bloor, M. (1997) 'Addressing social problems through qualitative research', in D. Silverman (ed.) *Qualitative Research: Theory, method and practice*, London: Sage.

Bragg, S. (2007) '"Student Voice" and governmentality: the production of enterprising subjects?', *Discourse: Studies in the Cultural Politics of Education*, 28 (3): 343–358.

Cahill, C. (2004) 'Defying gravity? Raising consciousness through collective research', *Children's Geographies*, 2 (2): 273–286.

Cahill, C. (2007) 'Doing research with young people: participatory research and the rituals of collective work', *Children's Geographies*, 5 (3): 297–312.

Carr, W. and Kemmis, S. (1986) *Becoming Critical: Education, knowledge, and action research*, London: Falmer Press.

Edwards, R. and Mauthner, M. (2002) 'Ethics and feminist research: theory and practice', in M. Mauthner, J. Jessop and T. Miller (eds) *Ethics in Qualitative Research*, London: Sage.

Frisby, W., Maguire, P. and Reid, C. (2009) 'The "f" word has everything to do with it: how feminist theories inform action research', *Action Research*, 7 (1): 13–19.

Geertz, C. (ed.) (1973) 'Thick description: toward an interpretive theory of culture', in *The Interpretation of Cultures: Selected essays*, New York: Basic Books.

Hart, R. (1992) *Children's Participation: From tokenism to citizenship*, Florence: UNICEF.

Heath, S., Brooks, R., Cleaver, E. and Ireland, E. (2009) *Researching Young People's Lives*, London: Sage.

Issitt, M. and Spence, J. (2005) 'Practitioner knowledge and the problem of evidence based research policy and practice', *Youth and Policy*, 88: 63–82.

Jarvis, P. (1999) *The Practitioner-Researcher: Developing theory from practice*, New York: John Wiley and Sons.

Lewin, K. (1948) *Resolving Social Conflicts: Selected papers on group dynamics*, ed. Gertrude W. Lewin, New York: Harper and Row.

LLUK (2010) *National Occupational Standards for Youth Work*, at: http://www.lluk.org/wp-content/uploads/2010/11/National-Occupational-Standards-for-Youth-Work.pdf (accessed 2 January 2011).

McCulloch, K. (2009) 'Ethics, accountability and the shaping of youth work practice', in R. Harrison, C. Benjamin, S. Curran and R. Hunter (eds) *Leading Work with Young People*, London: Sage/Open University Press.

McLeod, J. (1999) *Practitioner Research in Counselling*, London: Sage.

McWilliam, E. (2004) 'W(hi)ther practitioner research?', *Australian Educational Researcher*, 31 (2): 113–126.

Middleton, E. (2006) 'Youth participation in the UK: bureaucratic disaster or triumph of child rights?', *Children, Youth and Environment*, 16 (2): 180–190.

Perryman, J. (2006) 'Panoptic performativity and school inspection regimes: disciplinary mechanisms and life under special measures', *Journal of Education Policy*, 21 (2): 147–161.

Rapoport, R. (1970) 'Three dilemmas in action research', *Human Relations*, 23 (6): 499–513.

Robson, C. (1993) *Real World Research: A resource for social scientists and practitioner-researchers*, Oxford: Blackwell.

Shaw, I. (2005) 'Practitioner research: evidence or critique?', *British Journal of Social Work*, 35: 1231–1248.

Sikes, P. and Potts, A. (eds) (2008) 'Introduction: what are we talking about and why', in *Researching Education from the Inside: Investigations from within*, London: Routledge.

Smith, M. (1999) *Praxis*, at http://www.infed.org/biblio/b-praxis.htm (accessed 9 July 2010).

Smith, M.K. (2007) 'Action research', in *The Encyclopaedia of Informal Education*, at: http://www.infed.org/research/b-actres.htm (accessed 30 November 2010).

Stanley, L. and Wise, S. (1993) *Breaking out Again: Feminist ontology and epistemology*, London: Routledge.

West, A. (1999) 'Young people as researchers: ethical issues in participatory research', in S. Banks (ed.) *Ethical Issues in Youth Work*, London: Routledge.

# Getting started

## Developing and designing research for practice

Stan Tucker

## Overview

I have had numerous conversations with students and practitioners hoping to use a small-scale research project as a means of exploring a particular policy or practice issue. Sometimes the motivation has been to gain a better understanding of what makes an organisation 'tick'. At other times the ambition has been to solve a problem or gain a clearer understanding of why people behave in the way that they do. However, a common feature of these conversations has been the desire to extend knowledge and understanding, improve skills and competence, and delve and dig into things that are sometimes taken for granted. At the same time the desire to produce a good-quality research project has generated a series of important questions:

- 'How do I get started?'
- 'What can I hope to achieve through a small-scale project?'
- 'How do I go about designing and producing a good research project that will stand up to scrutiny?'

This chapter aims to answer all of these questions. Designing good research is a skilled process that involves careful planning, the setting of clear aims, objectives and boundaries, and the selection of an approach and methods of investigation that are likely to generate reliable research data. The chapter, then, has a number of learning outcomes attached to it. You should critically reflect on these as you read through it. The outcomes are intended to:

- provide you with an understanding of how the process of research design can guide and support the generation of good-quality research
- support you in identifying and developing questions and hypotheses that directly relate to the aims and objectives of the research
- assist you in identifying and exploring appropriate academic literature that will support the process of research design

- help you identify and manage issues and problems that might occur when carrying out small-scale research
- assist you in exploring both the possibilities and limitations of small-scale research projects and their potential to have an impact on policy and practice.

It is important at this stage to begin to think about the kinds of issues you might like to explore in your day-to-day work with young people. Pause for a moment and reflect on the one issue that is currently dominating your thinking and how some form of research might help improve your knowledge, understanding or confidence to intervene in a different way. Hang on to that idea (it might be worth writing some short notes to clarify your thinking) as we will return to it towards the end of the chapter.

## A question of focus

It might seem obvious to say that any research project needs a clear focus. But this is an area where many individuals, groups and even organisations struggle to make sense of their research intentions. Let us take one specific area of work that attracts a great deal of attention in terms of youth work practice: risk. What do we mean when we talk about 'risk' in the lives of young people? Who is considered to be *at* risk and why? Is all risk potentially negative in terms of its outcomes or can some forms of risk be educative, inspirational and transformational? Does concern about risk merely 'problematise' the lives of some young people (Griffin 1993) or, as Jeffs and Smith (1996: 12) argue, can it 'criminalise perfectly legal and acceptable behaviour'? The point being made here is that the subject of risk is an enormous one that cannot be explored through the generation of one simple question. To make sense of the issue we have to define the scope of our interest (and that might change over time). We need to pin down what we actually want to find out and why. We need to clarify why we want to explore the issue and what we hope to learn.

For example, I recently went along to a presentation on the benefits of outdoor education. The speaker talked extremely enthusiastically about the risks and benefits attached to this form of education. Yet, he presented little information on young people's perceptions of either the risks or the benefits involved; the view presented was essentially an adult/expert one. I wanted to know much more about the perceptions of those young people who participate in such activities. At that point, I could have chosen to take my curiosity further in terms of developing a small-scale research project to try to explore young people's views. My preliminary research question might have been: 'What are young people's perceptions of the risks and benefits associated with outdoor education?' My intention in formulating the question in such a way is that it would give me a starting point for my research.

McNiff *et al.* (1996: 36) provide a very useful set of questions that need to be taken into consideration when developing research. Their particular interest in generating the questions relates to the development of good-quality action research but the questions posed are relevant to all small-scale research projects. The questions, in modified form (and with some more added), are presented in Box 2.1 for consideration.

## Box 2.1  Key questions for focusing research

- What is your research focus?
- Why have you chosen this issue as a focus?
- What kind of evidence can you produce to show this is happening?
- What can you do about what you find?
- Do you intend to explore the topic and increase knowledge and understanding and/or move towards some form of action to bring about change?
- How will you collect and collate your findings?
- How will you evaluate the outcomes/impact of your research?
- How will you ensure that any judgements you might make are reasonably fair and accurate and based on evidence?
- How do you intend to report your findings?

Take your time to read through the questions carefully. They should begin to suggest the possible shape of any research design process. We will pick up on the key issues raised as the chapter develops. By asking such questions, it is intended that the scope and aims of any research project will become clearer.

Before moving on to discuss the formulation of particular research questions in more detail, there is a need to determine the nature of small-scale research investigation. We have already begun to explore issues of focus and the way that narrowing the scope of any research investigation will be helpful. But there are other factors to consider when undertaking a small-scale research activity. It is also important to stress that small scale does not mean insignificant or irrelevant research. It is merely helpful in marking out the nature of the research activity. Much of the work of Bassey (1999) looks at how case studies can be used to explore the kind of situations in which individuals and groups might routinely find themselves – at work, in meetings, in small group situations, and so on. It also focuses on how such a methodological approach can help us to understand particular kinds of intervention, ways of working and professional practices. You will find a more detailed discussion later in the chapter about case studies themselves, but at this stage the main point to bear in mind is that such an approach has the potential to support the development of well-focused, small-scale research design.

## Practice-based task 2.1  Research topics

Reflect back on the issues raised so far about the importance of developing a research design that has a clear focus. Think about how the use of a case study might assist you in selecting a suitable topic for research. Then make a list of the research topics that could potentially lend themselves to this approach.

*Comment:* What did you cover in your list? Perhaps you wrote something about the value of exploring group work approaches with young people. Or noted down the possibility of evaluating a particular aspect of the work of your service – for example, the provision of advice on education and training. I went back to my earlier research question and pondered how I might, in focusing on young people's perceptions, ensure that I paid specific attention to the ways in which issues of risk and benefit are actually defined. I began the process of modifying and reformulating my original idea. This is an important aspect of research design and development. You might start with what I describe as a *working question* that is subsequently modified and perhaps changed as your thinking develops.

There are other factors that may well influence the scope of your research, and it is important to be realistic and reflect on these carefully. In Box 2.2 you will find a list of factors that need to be considered as you develop your thinking about the nature of a small-scale research project.

---

### Box 2.2  Factors to consider in research design

- The time you have available for the research.
- Your ability to gain access to a suitable setting or site for the research – and whose permission you might need to secure to work there.
- Research participants and their availability – young people, service managers, other workers, etc.
- Documents you might want to access to support your research – reports, policies, etc.
- How you are going to fit in all the tasks required – meetings, interviews, collating findings, etc.
- Ethical approval for your work, particularly when it involves young people or vulnerable individuals and groups.

---

The list is not intended to be exhaustive but hopefully it gives you a real sense of the variety of tasks that need to be considered as part of any research design process. The discussion now considers the issue of developing good-quality research questions in more detail.

## Research questions and hypotheses

For academically focused research to be defined as such, it has to be informed and shaped by a particular research question (or set of questions) or hypothesis. The question(s) or hypothesis provides the focus and context for all that follows: the methodology employed; the methods used; the data gathered; the findings and analysis; and the conclusions drawn. You will have noticed the introduction of a new term in this section – *hypothesis*. Obviously, then, it is important to define what we mean when we use this term in a research context. The next task has been developed to assist you in doing that.

## Practice-based task 2.2  Research questions and hypotheses

There are three parts to this task. The first part asks you to reflect on what constitutes a good-quality research question. The second part explores the concept of a hypothesis. In the final part we focus on some research questions and hypotheses in order to assess their effectiveness.

### Part 1

To begin with, write down what you think are the key characteristics of a good research question.

*Comment:* A research question needs to be 'answerable' in the sense that it can be explored and examined in a structured and systematic way. However, that is not to say that the question will necessarily be answered in any *absolute* sense. In exploring a research question you will hopefully gain new knowledge and understanding. At the same time you are also likely to raise issues, problems or concerns that require further investigation (sometimes through the development of a new research project). The wording of the question, therefore, has to be as clear and concise as possible. This requires the use of words that explain in the simplest way possible the intended *focus* of the research. Vague or poorly structured research questions invariably generate a strong sense of frustration on the part of the researcher and can lead to the production of unfocused and even irrelevant data.

### Part 2

Look at the definition of hypotheses presented by Bowling (2002: 120):

> With deductive reasoning the investigator starts with general ideas and develops a theory and testable hypotheses from it. The hypotheses are then tested by gathering and analysing data. In contrast, inductive reasoning begins with observations and builds up ideas and more general statements and testable hypotheses from them for further testing on the basis of further observations.

Now determine what marks out hypotheses as different from research questions.

*Comment:* You get a real sense from Bowling's definition of both the nature of hypotheses and how they are constructed. Clearly, hypotheses are used to aid the development of theories. They take the form of testable statements that can be confirmed or rejected on the basis of evidence. Notice also the different approaches to hypothesis building that can be taken. Deductive hypotheses are based on general ideas (theories, for example) that are subsequently tested, whereas inductive hypotheses are built through observations which lead to the development of theory. Did you find yourself reflecting on the way hypotheses seem to have roots more firmly grounded in scientific methods of investigation? Cohen *et al.* (2002) point towards the way that hypotheses are constructed using 'variables' that are presumed to have some kind of relationship to each other and that the relationship can then be tested. In adopting such a position it could be argued, for example, that human behaviour 'is a reaction to external stimuli and that it is possible to observe and measure it' (Bowling 2002: 119). Space does not permit me to explore this issue in more depth and it might be an area where you want to read more for yourself. The important point is that whether you use research questions or hypotheses, they will impact on the research design processes.

## Part 3

Have a look at the research questions and hypotheses outlined below. Make notes on which you think are strong and which are weak, and why.

1   Group work is a good way to promote social change.
2   The individual stages of social group work combine to support critical self-evaluation and personal change.
3   How can social group work be used as a tool for promoting self-evaluation and personal change in young people?
4   Can group work help young people develop?

*Comment:* In examining and reviewing the statements, it no doubt became apparent which are strong and which are weak, and why. If we take statements 2 and 3, for example, the direction and intentions of the research are self-evident. The focus on self-evaluation and personal change is specific. Statement 2 also makes it clear that there will be a need to look at the individual stages of social group work in order to explore its use. Statements 1 and 4 are much more vague in terms of focus and the intentions of any research work subsequently required. Some people, it should be pointed out, favour what they see to be the more rigorous 'fact-finding' intentions of hypothesis formulation and investigation. In essence, as Giddens (1975) asserts, a *positivist* position is adopted, with the social scientist acting in the role of the analyst, the formulator of theories, rules, and so on. Others are drawn towards a more *interpretivist* position and the opportunity to explore lived experience. Beck (1979: 141) for example, argues that 'the purpose of social science is to understand social reality as different people see it and to demonstrate how their views shape the action which they take within that reality'. (You will find further discussion of the distinction between these approaches in Chapter 9.) Whatever position you ultimately choose to adopt, the actual development of specific research questions and hypotheses can feel like a fairly long and drawn-out process at first – particularly when you are itching to get started. However, it is important at that stage to remember that, for a research project to have any chance of success, its focus has to be clear and well articulated.

## The issue of background and context

Having decided on the focus of the research project and articulated an appropriate research question or hypothesis, the next part of the research design process requires you to explore some of the background issues that might have a direct impact on your study. At one level you are creating the *preliminary context* that will guide your future research activity. At another you are beginning the process of *immersing yourself* in your chosen topic of study. Clearly there is a need to do some substantial background reading. For example, you might want to look at particular policies, or read articles in professional publications that include aspects of your proposed research topic. The development of a preliminary literature review can also be extremely useful. As Fink (2005) notes, this can be achieved through the exploration of appropriate academic texts, journals, online publications, and so on. At this stage the intention is to collect, collate and synthesise materials that might ultimately have an impact on and help frame your study. You need to guide the shape of your review through constant reference to your research question(s) or hypothesis.

There is much to be gained through reviewing the literature in your research area. You are likely to engage, or perhaps re-engage, with key theories and perspectives that influence practice. A look at relevant academic books and journals will help in discovering what is currently being written in your chosen area. You will be able to come to a view about what gaps appear to exist in current knowledge and how your work might contribute to extending professional and academic understanding. Research-focused journal articles and books often contain summaries of key literature, and they will introduce you to various methodological approaches to research that can assist you in formulating your own approach. Good research publications encourage a level of critical evaluation of research methodologies and methods that will help you to assess their potential relevance and value to your work.

Another important thing to do is talk about your research design ideas. You should engage with a variety of people who might be helpful in the process. Clearly, if you are studying for an academic qualification, then securing the support of an academic tutor will be crucial. They should be able to offer critical guidance and point you towards a range of appropriate texts. You can share and receive feedback on your research questions and explore the key aims and objectives of your research project. Work colleagues can help to generate a level of critical reflection and they are likely to understand and share the personal and professional motivations for your proposed work. If you are a practitioner (a youth worker or Connexions PA, for example), you might want to talk to your line manager, particularly if you need to negotiate time to carry out the research or perhaps gain permission to use a particular setting, place or group. At this stage you might also want to engage with young people to discuss your ideas and ascertain how they could be involved in aspects of your work – as both participants and 'co-inquirers' (see Fraser *et al.* (2004) for further discussion).

## Methodologies and methods

We now arrive at the point where we begin to explore specific aspects of how the research is going to be carried out. We shall look at matters concerned with *methodology* and *methods*. Methodological issues are concerned with the overall approach to be adopted within the research, whereas our discussion of methods covers the way in which the research is to be carried out.

Let us start with the question of methodology. I shall specifically focus on the case study methodology (Bassey 1999) to illustrate the points I wish to make here. (As you read through the book you will see that other methodologies are discussed in detail.) Let us start by trying to answer the question of why consideration of the methodological approach is such an important aspect of research design. I would argue that any methodology needs to be 'fit for purpose' – at a philosophical and a practical level. The case study approach permits a high level of interpretive analysis. It is designed to allow exploration of the day-to-day lived experiences of the participants. Emphasis is placed on gaining a sense of reality from the perspectives of those involved. Situations are looked at in the round and the approach allows for in-depth analysis of specific circumstances, interventions, ways of working, and so on. Those who work in this area would also claim that their work provides easily accessible accounts and access to complex and situated behaviours (Cohen *et al.* 2002). Different kinds of case study can be designed and developed, as you can see in Practice-based task 2.3. The important point is to decide which is most 'fit for purpose'.

### Practice-based task 2.3  Different case studies

First, I want you to read a quote from Brewer (2002: 76–77) below. When you have done that, write down the kinds of case study investigation you might carry out in a youth work practice context under each of the headings.

Stake (1998: 88–89) identified three different types of case study. The intrinsic case is the study of one particular instance (or perhaps the only instance) of the phenomenon because it is interesting in its own right; the instrumental case is studied because it facilitates understanding of something else, whether it be theoretical debate or a social problem; and the collective case studies several instances of the same phenomenon to identify common characteristics.

In Box 2.3 I have listed my thoughts about the kinds of research activity that might be relevant using the three categories outlined in the quote from Brewer.

---

## Box 2.3  Research activities

| *Intrinsic case study* | *Instrumental case study* | *Collective case study* |
|---|---|---|
| Telephone counselling service for young people.<br><br>Local street work project. | Rough sleeping – to gain an understanding of homelessness issues.<br><br>Work of local youth council – to explore participation and democracy. | Review of youth arts provision in voluntary and statutory sectors.<br><br>Implementation of participation policy in a local authority youth service. |

---

Having decided on the methodological approach, it is then important to consider the research methods you might use to carry out your research project. With the case study approach you need to select those methods that reflect the intentions of such work. If you are not clear about the difference between methodology and method, look again at the definitions given earlier.

In selecting the methods you are going to use to collect data for your research there is a need to reflect carefully on how these methods will meet the requirements of your particular methodology. For the purposes of the discussion here, we are using the case study approach to illustrate the discussion. The *case study* is designed to allow the use of 'mixed methods' – those methods that are able to generate a range of data drawn from different sources (Bassey 1999). Case studies tend to produce what is sometimes described as 'thick description'. Geertz (1975) defines data like that as being 'rich' and possessing significant 'depth'. Its generation can be used to test ideas and theoretical perspectives. You will recall that case studies are intended to allow you to explore particular situations in which people might find themselves: forms of professional practice, various social arrangements, and so on. The 'thick description' produced is likely to be based on various conversations, social interactions, and so on. Therefore, the research methods employed need to be able to capture such forms of data. Two particular methods are highly relevant here – *interviews* and *observations*. Both of these methods will produce *qualitative* data: that is, data based on lived experience in terms of what can be seen and heard. For Denscombe (1998: 174), 'qualitative research relies on transforming information from observations, reports and recordings into data in the form of the written word, not numbers'. Clearly, things that people say and do are more likely to help us produce the kind of data described. It is also important to remember that it may be useful to collect other kinds of data. For example, we might want to look at the policy documents of a local youth centre to see if there is a connection between policy and practice. Or we may want to examine central or local government policies to see how youth counselling and advisory projects are justified, funded and evaluated. This form of activity is called 'documentary analysis' (Cohen *et al.* 2002: 147). It is important to remember that such documents may be unrepresentative, 'lack objectivity' or 'be deliberately deceptive'. As the researcher, you are likely to be using them in ways that were not originally intended. (Barker and Alldred discuss the use of documentary analysis in greater detail in Chapter 7.)

Finally, you might want to generate 'quantitative data', 'whose aim is to measure phenomena so that they can be transformed into numbers' (Denscombe 1998: 174). This might be achieved through the development of a questionnaire or survey. You could, for example, decide to survey users' opinions of a particular service provided in a youth centre.

Each of these methods is now explored briefly here (and each is discussed in more detail in later chapters).

*Interviews* are the most widely used research method employed in case study work (Bassey 1999). However, it is important that the design of the interview enables the researcher to gather appropriate data. The interview is a particular kind of conversation. It has a specific focus or purpose, which relates directly to your research question or hypothesis. You can employ several different kinds of interview. The *structured interview* consists of a set of predetermined questions to be asked of all participants in the research process. One of the main advantages of this approach is that a good level of consistency can be produced in terms of data collection and analysis through the use of the common questions. However, the rigid nature of the interview structure prevents the use of follow-up or additional questions and it can feel inflexible from the perspective of the researcher.

The *semi-structured interview*, on the other hand, can offer an increased level of flexibility. Here, a range of predetermined questions is also employed, but additional questions can be used to pursue a specific topic in more depth or to follow up an emergent theme or issue. However, it is important to acknowledge that there are inherent disadvantages with this method, too. The researcher can become side-tracked if too much time is taken following up specific lines of conversation. In addition, the flexibility offered through the questioning structure can make it difficult to categorise and analyse data.

The final kind of interview is the *unstructured interview*. This is perhaps the most difficult form of interview for the novice researcher to employ. As the name suggests, predetermined questions are not employed, and while the focus of the interview is determined in the normal way by the research question or hypothesis, a much more conversational style is used to facilitate interaction between the interviewer and interviewee. Such an approach obviously creates a high degree of flexibility and the possibility of exploring issues in great depth. However, it requires a high degree of skill in interviewing and the ability to stay focused in terms of the issue under investigation (see Denscombe (1998) for more detailed discussion).

Whatever interview method is ultimately chosen, the researcher is required to undertake some level of preliminary piloting (Cohen *et al.* 2002). Such activity normally requires the production of a draft interview schedule with appropriate questions. The purpose of the pilot is to test out both the approach to be adopted – for example, the semi-structured interview – and the wording and organisation of specific questions. Consideration needs to be given to the nature of the language used, whether the person acting in the interviewee role understood the questions and how they were organised and delivered. It is also possible to ascertain how long the interview might take to complete. Piloting often leads to a change in the structure and organisation of the interview. It is important to note that the piloting of all research methods is important. It gives you the opportunity to gauge whether the proposed method is likely to gather the kind of data you require, and it provides you with the opportunity to restructure or reorder your work.

Now, we move on to the issue of how the design of observation activities has to be built into the planning process. As with interviews, *observations* need to be 'fit for purpose'. If you want to use observations, you need to look at your interview questions or hypothesis and decide what value an observation will have in providing different kinds of data to that which you might gather through, say, interviews. The next short task should help you to think about this point.

## Practice-based task 2.4  Using observations

Reflect on the kinds of situation where it might be valuable to use observations when engaging in research work with young people. Write some short notes on why you think this method would be particularly useful.

Observations can be extremely useful for capturing the dynamics of a particular situation or exploring individual or group interactions. They can be used to study work practices or the outcomes of an intervention. They can be a powerful means of examining specific forms of behaviour as well as when and how they occur. I remember undertaking a small-scale piece of research that focused on the aggressive behaviour of a group of young men in a youth centre. I was keen to try to understand both what forms of behaviour were consistently displayed and the situations that had produced them. I had conducted some semi-structured interviews with the group concerned and gathered useful data on their individual and collective perceptions. In analysing the data

I noticed that a number of the participants raised the issue of the way the 'climate' in the centre changed when certain members of staff were working. I specifically used a number of observations to look at staff interactions with young people and the ways that they communicated. I was also interested to learn if particular situations or activities (among staff and young men) triggered aggressive forms of behaviour. You can see here how the use of a 'mixed methods' approach (Bassey 1999) proved important in generating different kinds of related data. In turn, the use of observations helped me to test out ideas that had been raised by the group of young people during the course of the interviews.

It is important to say that, as with interviews, observations can be used in different ways and for different purposes. In the example presented above, my observations were very specifically structured. I wanted to focus on specific forms of behaviour and how, or when, they manifested themselves. On other occasions I have used observations as a method of capturing the way in which a youth project is managed and run. I have focused on staff relationships and the way in which the work programme is organised and delivered, and have even observed meetings between staff and young people to increase understanding of how they relate to each other.

One of the major challenges facing the researcher when using observations is how to capture the data produced. The danger with observation is that *everything* becomes interesting! That is why it is important to give the observation a clear sense of purpose and relate it specifically to the intentions of the research project. You need to record the outcome of any observation carefully, which can be achieved by taking well-structured notes. You should write up an account of the observation as soon as possible after it has finished. It might be worth using a video camera to record a group activity. However, you must obtain the permission of the participants to do this. Cohen *et al.* (2002) provide a very detailed account of the nature of observational work and its potential advantages and disadvantages.

We shall now consider the use of *documents*. Any process of research design needs to pay attention to the documents it might be worth assembling to support the research activity. Documentary analysis (Denscombe 1998), as previously mentioned, can provide vital sources of information to assist you in understanding the background to a research issue. I analysed various documents when I undertook my work on trying to understand the aggressive behaviour of the group of young men in the youth centre. These included minutes of the centre management committee, where this issue had been discussed, daily recordings produced by the youth worker, and extracts from a 'centre log', in which notes were shared between members of staff. When using such data, however, it is important to remember that it has been produced for a variety of purposes not directly related to your research. As Hakim (2000) notes, we engage in a form of 'secondary analysis' with documents being drawn from two sources: 'primary sources' (documents generated during the period of the research) and 'secondary sources' that offer interpretations of events based on those primary sources.

Finally, let us reflect on the ways in which the development of a questionnaire survey might be used as part of the formulation of a research strategy. As with other research methods considered at the design stage, the questionnaire needs to be 'fit for purpose'. Questionnaires are useful for capturing data that can be expressed quantitatively or numerically. They are frequently used, for example, to gauge opinion or to rate a set of options or ideas. In the main, questionnaires are employed to explore the views of a cross-section of individuals and groups (Cohen *et al.* 2002). The questions employed tend to be 'closed', in that they require a definite response, such as 'yes' or 'no'. Or they might make use of a scale, such as the Likert scale (named after its author, Rensis Likert), to demonstrate a particular preference. It is also possible to include 'open' questions, where space is provided for respondents to express a view or opinion in their own words. As with other research methods, questionnaires require some level of piloting to ensure their quality. This normally involves reviewing the order of questions, their clarity, and crucially the time it takes to complete. It is important to remember when devising a questionnaire that people will have a limited amount of time for completion. Avoid, wherever possible, the use of technical language and complex or unnecessarily complicated questions.

In my experience, students are often drawn to the use of the questionnaire at the design stage of a research project. They see its potential in terms of reaching a wide audience and securing a strong cross-section of opinion. They are hopeful that people will want to complete the questionnaire and at the same time find it an interesting activity. Yet, several potential drawbacks in its use need to be carefully considered. Questionnaires can be costly to distribute, particularly if some form of postal activity is required. Sometimes they have to be distributed by a third party (such as the youth worker in a centre), and this can mean that control of the questionnaire is lost. Response rates are notoriously poor (depending on the subject and the target group), and it can be difficult to analyse the opinions provided through open questions (Bell 2005). Such factors need to be carefully considered before a decision is made to spend time developing a questionnaire.

## Designing in quality

In this section, I want to discuss four key concepts that will support you in producing high-quality research. Each of the areas needs to be carefully considered at the design stage. The four areas are: ethical considerations, triangulation, validity and reliability.

Although research ethics are discussed in detail in Chapter 3, it is important to set them in the context of research design. So, when we talk about the *ethical considerations* involved in research design, what do we mean? In order to answer this question, Oliver (2004) explores some of the key issues that need to be examined in approaching research design. The reasons for avoiding any kind of research that might 'damage' potential participants are debated. The principle of obtaining 'informed consent' from participants is discussed. The need to consider both the requirements and potential benefits for those taking part is considered. Thought is also given to how research work involving 'vulnerable individuals and groups' should be developed. Indeed, Oliver (2004: 9) specifically argues that 'it is important to consider [such] ethical issues from the early stages of a research project. From the beginning of the design process . . . to the methodology.' There is also a need to secure ethical permission to carry out research. This is generally obtained from a recognised local or national body, professional association or university research ethics committee. As part of the process of securing ethical approval, a formal application will normally need to be submitted.

## Practice-based task 2.5  Ethical principles for youth work

Write down a set of common principles that you believe should inform all research carried out by youth workers with young people.

Look carefully at the list you have created in Practice-based task 2.5. Does it protect the 'human rights' of all participants? Can those involved be confident of retaining their anonymity, confidentiality and the right to withdraw from the research process at any time? Does your set of principles guarantee that participants share the intentions of the research and the outcomes? What about the production of any final report or article? Do the participants have a role to play in its compilation or can they at least see a summary of the research? Did you find yourself thinking about who 'owns' research data and the need to record and reproduce those data as fairly and accurately as possible? Clearly, all of these matters should be considered when engaging in research design.

Let us move on now to the *triangulation* of research data, which again needs to be considered at the research design stage. Cohen *et al.* (2002: 112) provide a very useful definition of the process:

> Triangulation may be defined as the use of two or more methods of data collection in the study of some aspect of human behaviour . . . By analogy, triangulation techniques in the social sciences attempt to map out, or explain more fully, the richness and complexity of human behaviour by studying it from more than one standpoint, and in doing so, by making [possible] use of both qualitative and quantitative data.

From this definition, you can no doubt see how the process of triangulation is used to make links. In employing more than one method – such as interviews and observations – it is possible to compare and contrast data gained from different sources (as with my research on aggressive male behaviour in a youth centre). It moves research away from being 'single method' dependent, which can lead to bias or potential distortion of findings. It helps to build researcher confidence in the outcomes of the research where different methods provide a good level of data correlation. Again, you will find a more extensive discussion of types of triangulation in the work of Cohen *et al.* (2002).

The concept of triangulation can be directly linked to the question of the *validity* of the research. Validity is defined by Brewer (2002: 46) as 'the extent to which the data accurately reflect the phenomenon under study'. Cohen *et al.* (2002) speak of the need for data to be explored for its 'honesty', 'depth', 'richness' and so on, in order to help gauge its validity. A very useful framework for examining the subject of validity is provided by Bell (2005: 117), who makes specific reference to the work of Sapsford and Jupp (1996). Here, a link is made to the fact that the design of a research process has to be able to produce 'credible' conclusions. A connection is made between the methodological approach and methods, evidence generated, analysis and outcomes. Bell (2005: 118) encourages the researcher to 'ask yourself whether another researcher using your research instrument and asking similar factual questions would be likely to get the same or similar response' as a possible test for determining levels of validity and reliability.

The concept of *reliability*, when looking at specific research methods, is perhaps easier, but still important, to understand. A research instrument, such as an interview or an observation, has to have the capability of generating similar data from similar groups of respondents over a period of time (Cohen *et al.* 2002). This is where piloting (discussed earlier) of a specific method assumes a high degree of importance. The research method should be tested and retested as necessary, and in doing so its reliability is likely to be increased.

## Summarising the research design process

I shall now attempt to pull together the various aspects of the research design process in a coherent way. Figure 2.1 should help in this respect. Look at the figure for a few moments and try to recall some of the key issues that are involved at each stage.

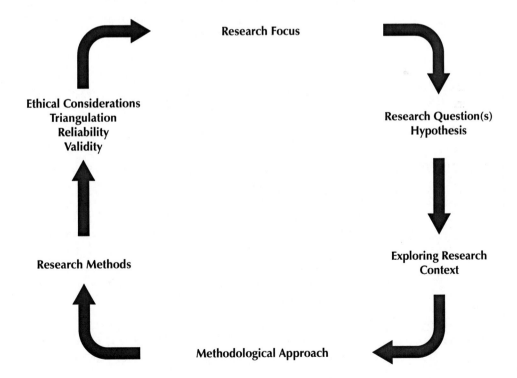

Figure 2.1 The research design process

You will no doubt recall at the beginning of the chapter that I devised a specific research question to help me explore young people's views on the risks and benefits of outdoor education. I now intend to use the research design process outlined above to reflect on some of the factors I would need to consider in taking such a study forward. I have done this in note form to demonstrate what would, in reality, be a very early stage in the overall design process. You will see the notes contain specific statements as well as questions that I need to address as the project develops. Although the notes refer to my original research question, a similar approach could be adopted to explore other issues and/or problems. You are asked to reflect on this point in Practice-based task 2.6.

---

# Box 2.4  Initial reflections on research design

| *Stages in research design focus* | *Factors to consider* |
|---|---|
| Research focus | Stimulated by attendance at presentation of research findings. Academic and professional audience. Questioned the absence of young people's views in case study approach adopted. Voices of young people vital in understanding how the value of such programmes is understood and evaluated. Small-scale research study seems appropriate in terms of capturing the voice of young people. |
| Research question | Formulation of a 'working question' to support the development of the design process. Acknowledgement of the fact that the question may need further refinement. Provides a starting point in relation to focus. Working question: 'What are young people's perceptions of the risks and benefits associated with outdoor education?' |
| Exploring research context | Need to seek out appropriate academic literature on outdoor education and informal education-related work. What national and local policy documents exist on outdoor education that need reviewing? Contact local youth service to see what work they undertake in this area. Undertake a computer search of organisations providing outdoor education – YMCA/YWCA mentioned as possible contacts. Look at research literature concerning the involvement of young people in research. |
| Methodological approach | Needs to be 'fit for purpose' in relation to research question. Possibly focused on a specific organisation or youth service. Consideration given to case study approach |

| | |
|---|---|
| | or ethnography. Matters of scale and feasibility are important to consider. What time have I available to undertake the research? How will I locate young people to take part in the research? |
| Research methods | Use of semi-structured interviews and some level of documentary analysis. Would there be any advantages in developing a questionnaire to cover a large group of young people? |
| Designing in quality | Reflect on ethical considerations in the design process. Mixed methods approach? Avoid being single method dependent. Reflect on issues of triangulation. Piloting of research methods will be essential – how can this be achieved? What about issues of validity and reliability? Build these into the overall design. |

## Practice-based task 2.6  Research design

At the start of the chapter you were asked to think about a possible research topic you might want to pursue. At this point I want you to write a set of notes, similar to those presented above, that will help you begin to explore some of the key issues and questions. Use the table format already provided.

I hope you find this a helpful approach. You need to undertake this kind of activity from a very early stage in the design of any research project. It will help you clarify your thoughts and come to a decision as to whether the research is feasible. You may need to rethink or modify your initial research question. You might find you spend a significant amount of time deciding on the focus. Understanding why you are motivated to undertake a specific research project is really important. Issues concerning the use of an appropriate methodology and methods will always take time to resolve.

## Summary points

- The process of research design is just as important as carrying out the research itself. If you invest time in producing a well-thought-out design you are much more likely to produce a strong research project that can stand up to scrutiny. The issue of scrutiny is an important one to consider. Those reading your research will not only want to explore the outcomes or data. They will also want to know *how* you produced that data and what motivated you to undertake the research in the first place. Some people will, rightly, want to study your methodology closely in relation to the claims you make for your work.

- Research should form a central aspect of work with young people. It should help to inform the development of policy and practice. The ability to generate good-quality research is essential to the management of good service provision. Indeed, there are increasing calls for young people to be directly involved in carrying out research themselves. Fraser *et al.* (2004) provide an excellent overview of this kind of work if you want to read further about 'doing research with children and young people'. Research design will help you to develop your planning and critical thinking skills. It also provides you with the opportunity to feel empowered, inquisitive and challenged.

## References and further reading

Bassey, M. (1999) *Case Study Research in Educational Settings*, Buckingham: Open University Press.

Beck, R.N. (1979) *Handbook in Social Philosophy*, New York: Macmillan.

Bell, J. (2005) *Doing your Research Project: A guide for first-time researchers in education, health and social care*, Maidenhead: Open University Press.

Bowling, A. (2002) *Research Methods in Health, Investigating Health and Health Services*, Buckingham: Open University Press.

Brewer, J.D. (2002) *Ethnography*, Buckingham: Open University Press.

Cohen, L., Manion, L. and Morrison, K. (2002) *Research Methods in Education*, 5th edition, London: Routledge Falmer.

Denscombe, M. (1998) *The Good Research Guide for Small-Scale Social Research Projects*, Buckingham: Open University Press.

Fink, A. (2005) *Conducting Research Literature Reviews from the Internet to Paper*, 2nd edition, London: Sage.

Fraser, S. Lewis, V. Ding, S. Kellett, M. and Robinson, C. (2004) *Doing Research with Children and Young People*, London: Sage.

Geertz, C. (1975) *The Interpretation of Cultures*, London: Hutchinson.

Giddens, A. (1975) *Central Problems in Social Theory*, London: Macmillan.

Griffin, C. (1993) *Representations of Youth: The study of youth and adolescence in Britain and America*, Cambridge: Polity Press.

Hakim, C. (2000) *Research Design*, 2nd edition, London: Routledge.

Jeffs, T. and Smith, M.K. (1996) '"Getting the dirtbags off the streets" – curfews and other solutions to juvenile crime', *Youth and Policy*, 52: 1–14.

McNiff, J., Lomax, P. and Whitehead, J. (1996) *You and Your Action Research Project*, London: Hyde.

Oliver, P. (2004) *The Student's Guide to Research Ethics*, Maidenhead: Open University Press.

Sapsford, R. and Jupp, V. (eds) (1996) *Data Collection and Analysis*, London: Sage.

Stake, R. (1998) 'Case studies', in N. Denzin and Y. Lincoln (eds) *Strategies of Qualitative Inquiry*. London: Sage.

# 3 Research ethics

## Participation, social difference and informed consent

Chrissie Rogers and Geeta Ludhra

## Overview

This chapter, as the title suggests, is about research ethics. But unlike many books on this subject, we have attempted to move beyond simply 'how to do' research ethically. Our aim is to aid the youth practitioner-researcher in thinking through ethical issues. Thus, as some of the more obvious questions about confidentiality, honesty, integrity and 'acting within the law' are addressed in other works (Wilson 2009: 66), we have used the space to explore more specific ethical issues.

In this chapter we will introduce ethics in its broadest sense and further discuss its position in terms of social difference (or *intersectionality*). Throughout the chapter, we will address challenges, opportunities and constraints of 'doing ethical research' and discuss these in relation to voice, informed consent, participation and research roles. 'Voice' and 'informed consent' will be covered through discussion relating to current research. 'Participation and research roles' will be exemplified through our studies and examples from international research. These four areas have ethical dilemmas attached to them and all can challenge and constrain the research process. We take the view that sensitive research will pose challenges and ethical dilemmas, but it should be critically engaged with and not dismissed for 'safer' or easier alternatives. Such research offers valuable opportunities for representing marginalised views and young people's interpretations. Some broad questions related to this include:

- Whose voice is narrated throughout the research? The young person's or the researcher's?
- Who consents to the research? The young person or the gatekeeper?
- How *included* in the *whole* research process (from design to analysis) is the young person?
- What role does the researcher play in the life of the young person and how does that relationship develop? Is the researcher a friend, a counsellor or an 'objective' observer?

None of these questions has a simple answer, as each research context is unique. To support the researcher in this process, we have posed reflective questions throughout the chapter. But in one section we take this a step further by drawing on our own research experiences: we put forward cases as examples, suggesting ways of engaging with ethics at a more practical level. Finally, we provide a summary with suggestions for further reading. As there are many books in this area, we hope the references and research cited throughout the chapter will also support additional reading.

## Context: what is research ethics?

In the UK, social science research generally requires ethical approval when involving children and young people (BSA 2004; BERA 2004). In this case, what can *really* be understood by the phrase 'doing ethical research' and what claims can be made in addressing ethics for the purpose of exploring 'new' knowledge around the lives of young people? Young people are not a homogeneous group, so researchers cannot claim that they are. It is important to understand early on in the process of 'doing ethical research' that young people are involved in change making and indeed want to be (Weller 2007a, 2007b). But still, huge numbers of young people are excluded from being heard or represented in different ways across different countries (Gillies and Robinson 2010a, 2010b). This is an ethical issue in itself.

In terms of getting young people involved in research and therefore seeing them as social actors, the New Social Studies of Childhood (NSSC) has positively responded to this concern. Children, and indeed young people, have become increasingly acknowledged as agents of change; as 'competent social actors' (Barker and Weller 2003b: 207; Barker and Smith 2001). In rethinking how we explore the experiences of children and young people, Kellet (2010: 7) quite rightly posits the need to shift our thinking as researchers from researching 'on' children to researching 'with' children and to expand this framework to research 'by' children. Politically, within the UK, various pieces of legislation, such as the Children Act (1989) and Every Child Matters: Change for Children (2004), have been important in laying foundations, as have other political directives and documents. The Every Child Matters agenda sets out changes in ways that support and care for children and young people. There are five categories in the agenda, but one in particular suggests children and young people should be empowered to make a positive contribution to society – hence 'inclusive' and participatory research feeds comfortably into this agenda. In addition, the ten-year youth strategy (DCSF 2007) schemes aim to empower young people (Heath *et al.* 2009).[1]

Moreover, in thinking about how children and young people should be involved and represented in research, an engagement with issues surrounding diversity and difference is essential. As already suggested, young people are not a homogeneous group, so attention to 'difference' is vital. Innovative and participatory methodologies (as in Sutton *et al.* 2007) are beginning to account for the inclusion of marginalised and vulnerable young people so that their voices become central in government policy agendas. Such methodologies carve valuable spaces and opportunities for them to analyse and reflect upon their own situations and suggest strategies for tackling such issues as poverty (Bennett and Roberts 2004). Heath *et al.* (2009: 42) discuss notions of 'sameness' and 'difference' as important issues in ethics and research with young people. They emphasise how an understanding of these factors can eliminate 'taken for granted' assumptions. In relation to power differences between adult researchers and young people, it is clearly more ethical to represent the marginalised positions of young people in central policies, as they are the ones who are directly influenced.

Differences may include social class (even caste), ethnicity, religion, disability, sexuality, gender, age, mental health, and so on. The list is endless, with some of these factors intersecting in complex, overlapping ways. Aapola *et al.* (2005) highlight how culture, ethnicity, religion and social class impact on differing attitudes and generational practices within families in relation to the upbringing of children. Differences may be seen in how young people access different resources (cultural, religious, economic and social) within their family and social contexts. These impact on the choices and opportunities available to young people, and the conditions of access and support are further determined by internal psychological factors and different degrees of agency that individuals express.

In this way, researchers must critically reflect on social differences and the ways in which some young people may face simultaneous axes of oppression (Gillborn and Youdell 2009; Mirza, 2009). In exploring these differences, it is important to engage with ethically orientated questions which require an understanding and sensitivity of a particular sample's unique needs (e.g. disabled children, black or South Asian young women). We could question, for example:

- What does 'social difference' actually mean to a young adolescent girl of working-class Bengali origin? How could a youth practitioner-researcher access her views?
- What are the ethical considerations required for accessing the views of young adolescent girls of working-class Bengali origin?
- What are the ethical considerations required for adolescent boys on the autistic spectrum? How can a youth practitioner-researcher engage in research whereby their interpretations and the young person's voice are accurately represented without being stereotyped or homogenised within other groups?

Thinking about ethics at the beginning of the research process or simply completing an ethics form does not constitute 'critical engagement' (Miller and Bell 2002; Liamputtong 2007). Feminist researchers have influenced the debates around ethical research, as has disability research more recently. Feminists, as researchers (and we include ourselves here), contend that knowledge is 'grounded in individual and collective experiences and this means that the course of a project may only be guessed at initially' (Miller and Bell 2002: 34; Liamputtong 2007; Mirza 2009). Crucially, discussing what the research might achieve in its aims and objectives and informing participants of this are not reflections on what the outcomes become over the course of collecting and analysing data. Of course, engaging with participatory research (discussed below) might well overcome or diffuse some of the challenges related to 'doing ethical research', but we must ask *whether it is always possible or appropriate to do such research*.

Going a step further and claiming to 'empower' and 'give voice' to research participants in an emancipatory way is naive and simplistic (Swartz 2011) as each individual and research interaction is unique. In line with postmodern theory, 'mini-narratives' offer valuable insights into specific cultural and social contexts (Liamputtong 2007), but this does not mean that such research can 'empower' large groups and this is not necessarily what social research aims to do; empowering is often about a small group of unique individuals. It is, however, in the transferability of those 'mini-narratives' or findings at wider policy level that broader impact can be made at national or international level.

## A critical discussion of ethics in relation to opportunities, challenges and constraints: voice and informed consent

We shall now discuss ethical dilemmas and outline opportunities, challenges and constraints facing both youth researchers and young research participants. As researchers, in the context of this chapter, we write from an 'insider' feminist perspective, and this raises important issues for the scrutiny of our own research positions, attitudes, beliefs and feelings through personal childhood history (Greene and Hogan 2005; Breen 2007). In doing so we acknowledge that we share some parallel experiences of young people's worlds through a connected identity and personal lived history. In undertaking our respective studies, we both recognise the role of the 'self' and are transparent about our research positions. In understanding the 'self' and the methodologies we adopt with the young people (and parents, in Chrissie's case), we have engaged in a process of reflexive writing (Hertz 1997; Alvesson and Skoldberg 2009) and dialogue so that the interactions between our participants and ourselves are critically questioned at multiple levels (Etherington 2009; Bridges 2009).

### *Ethical voice, ethical knowledge*

In thinking about representing young people's voices as an ethical challenge – and, indeed, an opportunity – Roberts (2008) suggests that asking children and young people questions has been going on for a long time. Voices from children were heard in the nineteenth century when, as paupers, their stories about emigration to Canada were reported. As one child said, 'We all sicked over each other' during the sea crossing; another, when asked about adoption, replied, ''Doption sir, is when folks gets a girl to work without wages' (Roberts 2008: 260). However, crucially, over decades children and young people have been silenced due to their assumed lack of knowledge and experience. Moreover, as Morrow and Richards (1996: 93) point out, much research in the twentieth century concentrated on *adult* views of children and young people, so much so that, even within education and the family (in which children and young people are embedded), studies missed the point and asked adults for *their* views on children and young people's lives. Importantly, though, if children and young people are willing to give their views on subjects about which they are, in a sense, experts – such as family life and education – we (in the broadest sense, including politicians, government departments, service providers and others) should be willing to listen to what they have to say, and incorporate their views into our understandings. Without asking children and young people for their views directly, it is all too easy to fall into imputing views to them, and stereotyping 'youth' on the basis of small samples or anecdotes (Roberts 2008: 270).

We are not suggesting here that adult participants' views and commentaries are unimportant; after all, we have all experienced childhood. But what must be appreciated are the different contexts and conditions of the twenty-first-century child, and how they, as children and young people, perceive, interpret and negotiate their lived experiences, rather than the researcher's interpretation of their lives (Kellet 2010). Participatory methods with young people, for example, provide valuable space for participants to 'define their own reality and challenge imposed knowledge' (Veale 2005: 253–254; see also Belenky *et al.* 1986). By researching in less restrictive ways, young people are ensured greater space to articulate their opinions at length (Connolly 1998; Alldred and Burman 2005). Therefore, whilst the challenges are significant, the opportunities are greater. But, as Cairns (2009) quite rightly points out, in engaging with the ethical dilemmas of 'voice', representation and ethics in discourses of youth literature, we often raise more questions than answers.

Woodhead and Faulkner (2008: 20) reveal that in the early 1970s, in laboratory-based psychological research, 'children were tantalised with a toy' which they were then told they could not touch. These children were observed and in some cases were punished 'with a loud noise or some other unpleasant experience' if they even attempted to touch the toy. This now seems utterly indefensible as the children were not asked to consent and inevitably underwent a distressing experience. Each child's voice was indeed unheard.

To move into more sociological research, we draw attention to a commonly cited piece of research (Humphreys 1970) that has been a source of ethical controversy when thinking about voice and indeed informed consent. Whilst this particular piece of research is not about young people, it is illuminating for different reasons from those in the aforementioned psychological research. Humphreys' participants were not in danger of physical or emotional pain, but still the research process was considered deeply unethical. Humphreys covertly participated (as a voyeur) in 'the tearoom trade'. 'The researched' were gay men who engaged in sexual activity in public toilets (the so-called tearooms). He recorded their activity via journal entries but also noted their vehicle number plates (and so was able to trace their addresses through a friend 'on the inside'). Later, he visited their homes in disguise as a market researcher. The research revealed that a number of the men engaging in gay sex in the tearooms were also in heterosexual relationships and had children.[2] Humphreys' work highlights the tension between the pursuit of knowledge and understanding about a particular phenomenon and potential participants' (individual) rights and liberty, which cut across age and any other social difference.

The research mentioned above draws attention to various challenges and constraints. For example:

- Whose voice is heard?
- How is the process of 'informed consent' and access to young people's voice negotiated ethically by the researcher before and throughout the research process?
- What questions can be asked and whose questions (or 'research agendas') are they?
- Can the researcher sensitively ask questions of a more emotional nature without causing distress or discomfort (see Humphreys 1970; Ludhra forthcoming)?

To summarise, 'doing ethical research' does not mean that we omit sensitive topics because we are worried about the consequences. This is simplistic and naive. As researchers, we also think within a 'moral framework' of ethics (see Wilson 2009: 66–67) and child-centred research practices offer genuine opportunities for young people to contribute their representations and worldviews. As Flick (2009) points out in a 'commonsense' notion, the researcher must consider the participants' perspectives at all times and any expectations made of them. Furthermore, a sense of 'humanness' and consideration of 'fairness' (Liamputtong 2007) for those involved is vital. Conducting research as 'you would be done by' is a sound guiding principle here (Sikes and Potts 2008: 8).

## Consenting to what?

Matters concerning 'informed consent' are continually discussed by researchers and often considered challenging. Naive assumptions that telling research participants the objectives of the research and all the associated 'facts' about the process equate to 'doing ethical research' can be misleading (David *et al.* 2001: 348). Furthermore, as Chase (1996: 57) rightly says, 'An informed consent form cannot possibly capture the dynamic processes of interpretation and authorship.' It might therefore be sensible to consider 'process consent' (Smythe and Murray 2000) or an 'ethics-as-process' framework whereby continual renegotiation takes place as unforeseen circumstances arise (Liamputtong 2007: 44). This is similar to what many researchers in the UK call 'negotiated consent' (Miller and Bell 2002).

Informed consent is usually associated with a consenting adult, due to the fact that it has been assumed that children and some young people are not fully competent to give informed consent, and this consent is based on the participant gaining information about the research and then making a decision to participate based on that information (Morrow and Richards 1996: 94). According to Smythe and Murray (2000: 313), it is not dramatically different in Canada, as their research council also suggests that informed consent is a process of coming to reach an agreement and not simply about signing a form. In thinking about the challenges of ethical research, it should be remembered that consent is always provisional (Thompson and Holland 2003: 241) and, as suggested, it should be negotiated and renegotiated (Miller and Bell 2002).

Thinking about the challenges of 'doing ethical research' and 'informed consent', surely competence depends on the topic of research, the context and the stated objectives? Maybe it cannot be just about chronological age or level of 'competence'. Look at 'inclusive research', for example, especially with marginalised or 'vulnerable' people (Gillies and Robinson 2010b; Walmsley and Johnson 2003; Liamputtong 2007). Aspects of competency have been addressed, but further work needs to be done regarding, for example, mental capacity to understand the research. Medical ethics and consent are problematic, especially when couched in medical and legal terminology and practice. What makes consent appropriate and understandable and therefore believable and useful? Is it all about Gillick competency (David *et al.* 2001: 349)?[3] For example, childhood research often focuses on gaining consent 'or allowing for dissent from being "empowered" through having their voices heard' (David *et al.* 2001: 349). It is important to note that we must not necessarily 'avoid asking the questions because they are ethically difficult, thereby excluding children from research is an ethical position in itself' (Morrow and Richards 1996: 103).

We cannot exclude certain 'groups' of young people – for example, intellectually disabled people, or those with mental health difficulties, or sex workers – merely because hearing their voices might be practically difficult or pose ethically challenging or disturbing dilemmas for the researcher. This is a challenge that youth practitioners face when working with young people and they must address such difficulties within an 'ethical' and moral framework that is specific to each unique context. This leads us to question whether researchers should consider terminating the research if unanticipated outcomes place research participants in danger (Smythe and Murray 2000). It would be sensible to say 'yes'. But to what degree can we predict the underlying impact and potential harm of the study or the researcher on the participant (see Goodson and Sikes 2001)? How can space be created within research processes for young people to articulate the potential impact of participation at each stage? This will provide opportunities for the participant to revisit what they have consented to and whether they feel comfortable with that. When faced with such complex questions, participatory or 'inclusive' research seems the most ethical. Moreover, such processes facilitate the articulation of new voices and add a genuine 'multi-voicedness' approach in the research literature (Moen 2006). In exploring the more challenging areas of young people's lives we, as researchers, often enter the 'dark corners' of their lived experiences and have a moral responsibility to illuminate the darkness to understand better what happens in those 'in-between' and often 'no-go' areas (Cahill 2004: 283).

On reflection, the researcher could pose some of the following questions:

- Does the research involve an agreement/ground rules between the researcher and participants?
- Who has the right to give consent? A parent or a gatekeeper, perhaps?
- Does the research involve participants who can give informed consent?
- How will you, as a researcher-practitioner, check that the research has been fully understood and therefore that the consent is meaningful?
- To what degree is consent renegotiated and explained throughout the research process?
- Are there opportunities for participants to withdraw or discuss their feelings about involvement at various stages of the research process?

In response to these questions and the above assumptions about voice and informed consent, it makes sense now to discuss how to facilitate participatory research and the related ethical issues.

## A critical discussion of ethics in relation to opportunities, challenges and constraints: participation, research relationships and roles

Here, we shall embed the challenges, constraints and opportunities in the research of others and our own. Therefore, our respective UK studies are presented within the contexts of parenting, children identified with 'special educational needs' and South Asian girls. We also draw upon examples of global research from an international perspective.

### Ethics in relation to participation in research

We draw your attention to the questions below when thinking about the challenges, constraints and power relations within research where participants adopt more collaborative roles:

- Who benefits from the research?
- What purpose does the research serve?
- Who is the audience for the research?

These are by no means 'new' questions, as Cahill (2004) points out. However, as highlighted by Keddie (2000), they are not asked enough during research with young people. Academic research should not simply be an 'exclusive conversation' between 'us' as researcher-practitioners about 'them' as participants (Cahill 2004: 282). Surely, this in itself is morally and ethically unsound and reduces the impact and readership of research.

Research that engages with young people's narratives and lived experiences can be overpowering and emotionally intrusive. Furthermore, the interpretation of the author can take a deeply personal experience away from the individual so that it becomes their interpretation of their life (Goodson and Sikes 2001; Clough 2002). Therefore, 'the assessment of "risk" in narrative research is a highly sensitive and idiosyncratic matter; one that resists any obvious formulation in terms of principles of minimal risk or uniform procedures for risk–benefit analysis' (Smythe and Murray 2000: 322).

When discussing participatory research in relation to ethics, it is meaningful to consider what participation really means and whether the researcher and participant see this in different ways? Does all ethical research have to be 'inclusive' and participatory, and is all 'inclusive' participatory research ethical or indeed emancipatory? 'Nothing about us without us' is commonly heard as a position statement within disability research (Walmsley and Johnson 2003). That is to say, some disabled people quite rightly say to researchers, 'Do not talk about our lives without asking *us* about *our* lives.' Ethical participatory research is about making sure that those young people participating in research are heard to the degree where their voices are integral to the narrative, both actually and analytically. To have young people involved in the research process is clearly challenging and time consuming but also full of opportunities as it offers windows into unique and alternative representations. It is here that we draw upon our own research experiences to highlight some of the opportunities and challenges.

In Geeta's Ph.D. research, her methodology engages with the research agendas of a group of South Asian girls (Ludhra and Chappell forthcoming). The literature in this area indicates that their everyday life experiences are hugely complex and multifaceted. The girls were encouraged to lead topics for discussion (the 'research agenda') and conversations opened with a 'generative narrative question' (Flick 2009: 177) to stimulate and frame the direction of the interview. Geeta posed an opening question: 'Talk to me about your identity and cultural experiences as an Asian girl. How do you experience life and who you are?' This exploration and focus on 'their' experiences through a series of three or four in-depth research conversations and reflective practices revealed how innovative and unique each girl's narrative was. For example, the girls reflected in diverse ways (all initiated by themselves). Reflections included pictorial analogies of identity, mind-maps, Post-it notes, magazine interpretations, e-mail reflections and discussions around holiday photographs. Engaging in such research as a young woman (or young person) is complex, requiring a deep level of self-reflection through a process that is facilitated through talk and metacognition (Evans and Jones 2009).

The girls, as young women, were examining and analysing intricate facets of their identity beyond description, and for many this was a first-time dialogue. They were asked for clarity, for example, on how they know and interpret what they explain and how school, family and friendships 'promote and hinder' their development and identities as young women (Belenky et al. 1986). Belenky et al. (1986: 4) highlight how the narratives of the American women in their study were 'catalytic in shaping the ways they viewed themselves' and those around them. In this way, such studies can be distressing but also empowering and emancipatory without necessarily planning for them to be so. Belenky et al. (1986: 4) describe this as 'the roar which lies on the other side of silence'.

Research with young people can be unpredictable and therefore it is often difficult to second-guess what will happen (Gillies and Robinson 2010a, 20010b). Also, there is the potential for loss of academic credibility (Smythe and Murray 2000: 321). In a climate that requires active researchers within higher education to contribute to high-impact and peer-reviewed journals, the voice of the participant as an active researcher is not always considered legitimate (Ludhra and Chappell forthcoming). In addition there can be a power divide in interpreting data (Heath et al. 2009: 66). However, critically involving young people early on may raise questions that were not considered by adult researchers, as innovative methodologies and practices often evolve over time and are not always planned. Kay's (2006) study with young Muslim girls in a participatory sports project revealed the benefit of involving them at the research stage, raising questions, conducting interviews and transcribing data from families by themselves. As a white female researcher, Kay realised the benefits of conducting research in this way in order to access particular views as an 'outsider'.

But including young people early on poses difficulties in terms of how funding often works, especially with respect to who pays (Kirby 2004: 14). Ultimately, participatory research is about *meaningful* participation (Kirby 2004), but questions can still be raised about when it becomes meaningful:

- Is it about bringing young people in from the beginning, during or at the end of the process?
- Are young researchers treated equally and with respect?
- In the end, will they benefit from the research and, if so, how is this explored or uncovered throughout?

(Ludhra and Chappell forthcoming)

Within ethical research, especially participatory research, power relationships are often discussed. It is assumed in much work that 'the researched' have little power or voice in the research process. But maybe it is not always the researcher who holds the power (Gillies and Robinson 2010a, 2010b). For instance, the gatekeeper might hold some power over the young person involved in the research. Geeta's Ph.D. research proved difficult in terms of gaining initial access to school settings, as school receptionists would sometimes withhold enquiries from senior staff, resulting in a lack of response to phone calls and e-mails. Access and trust were finally gained through academic research colleagues who 'paved the way' through personal contacts.

In considering this further, a youth work manager, for example, may well have gatekeeping access to a group of young people; a gang leader can have significant power over gang members; and school staff might hold some power within educational settings. It is important to explore and understand these power dimensions within the proposed research framework. Sometimes researchers might believe that gatekeepers give consent, but in reality it might only be that they open up access.

Therefore, which questions should a researcher pose when embarking on ethically sound participatory research?

- Does the research really address issues that matter to young people and will it lead to improved lives for them?
- Does the research genuinely represent the young people's lived experiences and views?
- Were the research questions identified by the young people or the researcher?
- Does the research enable the researcher and young people to work in collaboration?
- Is the youth practitioner-researcher on the side of the young person?
- Will the research be accessible to young people and, if so, how will the findings be disseminated?

These are important questions that researchers should ask before conducting participatory research (see Wilson 2009: 68–69). Of course, all the other ethical considerations still apply.

Such participatory research considerations feed into thinking ethically about research roles and relationships of power as participants become more involved in the study.

## Ethical research relationships and roles

Sometimes the relationships we develop with research participants are not considered as having any ethical implications, but in reality this aspect of the research process is crucial. What does the research relationship mean for the research participant, for the researcher or for the young people as co-researchers? What ethical boundaries or rules (Thompson and Holland 2003) are crossed, if any, if or when participants become friends? What is there to be gained from maintaining relationships?

For example, when Chrissie was carrying out her Ph.D. work, she was unsure of how to go about gaining access to mothers and fathers with children identified as having 'special educational needs'. However, her position as a mother with an intellectually disabled daughter meant that she already had particular parental networks. But was it ethical to use her personal contacts? Chrissie's contacts with some mothers of her daughter's peer group helped in accessing participants via the snowball method, but this source was not utilised to any great extent. In the main, she gained participants from the conferences she attended as both a researcher and a mother. Her 'insider' status facilitated this (Rogers 2003, 2007).

Both Geeta and Chrissie moved fluidly between their insider and outsider roles at different stages of the research process. This was often dependent on the relationship with each participant, the space in which they were researching, the topic and the context. In this way, their insider/outsider statuses were not fixed and at times they were 'incomplete' and 'unstable' (O'Connor 2004: 169). These positions sometimes drew on inner feelings and emotions, rather than on the physical persona of their identities. For example, during particular research experiences, Geeta's role was that of researcher in the school context. The content of some interviews often shifted her outsider status to insider as internal conversations were taking place that shifted the psychological frame of mind through a sense of connectedness.

Although Geeta had contacts through her two adolescent daughters and Asian female friendship networks, she decided not to draw on these insider links. For Geeta, the potential repercussions of what the young women might disclose about their extended family lives and how this might affect relationships with their parents were considered problematic at the time of planning the study. However, interactions with these young women (and women of her own age) on the inside have provoked additional thinking. For example, during the course of her research, Geeta has had deep internal conversations with the 'self'. This has also been the case for Chrissie. For example, after a parents' conference, on returning home in the evening, Chrissie was confused about her insider/outsider status. She questioned whether she was participating as a researcher or a parent. Such ethical issues raise complex challenges for the researcher yet open up valuable opportunities for new dialogues. As Oakley (1981: 58) points out, it is not easy *or necessary* to be uninvolved:

> It requires, further, that the mythology of 'hygienic' research with its accompanying mystification of the researcher and the researched as objective instruments of data production be replaced by the recognition that personal involvement is more than dangerous bias – it is the condition under which people come to know each other and to admit others into their lives.

Moreover, Adler and Adler (1997) discuss the challenges and opportunities of existing within different membership groups simultaneously: that of the parent member, the community member and the research member, effectively playing different roles and being seen as having those different roles by 'others'. In their longitudinal ethnographic study of 'children's worlds', they saw that the 'Overlap between researchers' personal lives and research role invoke methodological, epistemological and ethical issues salient to contemporary ethnographers.' They then suggested that 'the majority of the time we were able to integrate the research and the membership roles, engaging in them simultaneously' (Adler and Adler 1997: 26, 33).

Adler and Adler (1997) also found that their commitment to the parental membership status was stronger than other membership roles, and this at times impacted on them and those around them, both in the family and those 'being researched', and not always positively. Occasionally, they had to 'lose' participants due to their commitment to their parental role/membership. This is an ethical challenge in how to deal with the loss of participants and their data. In thinking further about ethics and roles, at the stage of the first interview, Chrissie was still under the illusion that she could separate her different roles. However, as the research progressed and as she reflected, it became clear that this was becoming increasingly difficult. Engaging with issues about the role of the researcher is crucial for both youth and education workers – 'researcher-practitioners' – who might be considered insiders, especially if the researcher is also a member of staff within a particular institution, or indeed if the group participating are part of the researcher-practitioner's community (Sikes and Potts 2008).

The idea of developing ethical research relationships could also be discussed in terms of the interview process. Provocatively, the unstructured interview has been recognised as 'seductive' in the same way as reality TV shows and 'true life' dramas are for avid fans (Silverman 2005: 344; Hey 2000). Furthermore, it has been accused of being too much like 'therapy'. However, the qualitative interview is neither a 'romanticized view of seamless authenticity emerging from narrative accounts' (Miller and Glassner 2004: 126) nor a counselling session for either the researcher or participants, and it must not be mistaken as such (Goodson and Sikes 2001).

Thus, with regards to developing an ethical relationship, Ellis and Bochner (2000: 754) ask:

> 'So what will you do if an interviewee breaks down or if you see a place where you could be of help?' She looks at me, waiting for the answer, then murmurs, 'I'm not sure.' 'What would you want someone in a similar situation to do for you if you were a research participant?' 'Well, I'd want them to understand where I was coming from . . . But isn't it true that not everybody can do good therapy? I mean most academics aren't trained therapists.'

Ellis and Bochner (2000) go on to explain that therapeutic training could be useful for the ethnographer, but that not everyone would be comfortable or able to deal with this sort of emotionality. Roberts (2008) discusses sharing information, and reminds us that to divulge an aspect of your 'self' in the research is unethical in recent history. But increasingly qualitative ethical research does not require the researcher to be removed emotionally. Chrissie, in her research journal, recalls this in relation to the potential development of relationships with research participants:

I'm halfway through the fieldwork process and the phone rings. 'Hello, is Chrissie there please?' 'Speaking,' I reply, not recognising the voice on the other end. 'It's Karen [pseudonym]. You interviewed me last year.' 'Oh, hi,' I replied, embarrassed that I hadn't immediately remembered her. 'I was wondering if you would like to meet for lunch to catch up?' she asked. 'Is everything OK?' I said, without really thinking. I thought perhaps she wanted to meet with me as my researcher self! Maybe there was something I could do for her, or maybe there was some more information about her son, who has Down's syndrome, that would be useful for the research? I was only half right. She did want to talk about her son but she wanted to 'catch up' as if we were old friends. We made an arrangement to meet at a local pub at a time that suited my already busy schedule. She wanted to know how my love life was, and what was going on in my daughter's life! I was touched by this but also concerned.

This situation clearly poses an ethical dilemma. What if all of Chrissie's participants wanted to 'catch up'? How would she deal with that? In reality, this was unlikely to happen, but at the time she remembers feeling concerned about her role in relation to the participants (a 'friend', perhaps?) and questioned who they were to her. As feminist researchers, both Chrissie and Geeta are in some way entwined in their personal narratives. For example, their identities draw on their practitioner, researcher and personal roles as mothers. The identities of other youth researcher-practitioners may also be connected with the young people they work with. Clearly, this raises ethical challenges; but as stated earlier, critical engagement with these positions through self-reflexivity is necessary if they are to make their viewpoints transparent (Liamputtong 2007; O'Connor 2004).

Geeta experienced periods of 'revisiting old ghosts' from the past as she engaged with the narratives of the young women she interviewed. At times this proved emotional and distressing. Moreover, Hertz (1997: xiii), in talking about 'reflexivity and voice', says, 'to make sense of what we observe or what people tell us, we may draw on the richness of our own experience, particularly if what we are studying we have also experienced. Parts of an interview may echo personal thoughts or prompt us to recall parts of our own lives.' Hence, it could be argued that being self-reflexive (O'Connor 2004) about the relationships that occur between the researcher and participants is critically ethical.

In summary, then, building ethical relationships is challenging but necessary. But that is not to say that all ethical research will engage in maintaining relationships in an in-depth way.

## A theoretical framework: principles for 'ethically responsible research'

We contextualise the practice-based tasks discussed below against a backdrop of four theoretically grounded principles for 'methodologically sound and ethically responsible research' (Gillies and Robinson 2010a: 100). We exemplify the four guiding principles posited by Gillies and Robinson that are gained from ethically challenging research with young people who were believed to have challenging behaviour. (In this chapter we are particularly interested in the first two. Principles 3 and 4 are more context specific, but are still important in certain situations.)

1  Explain the research clearly and carefully to gain pupils' informed consent.
2  Involve them in setting ground rules and planning sessions.
3  Avoid panicking and shifting between lots of activities in group sessions. Hold your nerve and persevere.
4  Ensure group activities are strategically targeted towards answering research questions.

(Gillies and Robinson 2010a: 100)

As said, these principles will not be appropriate for all research contexts; rather, they act as a valuable guide. Furthermore, they are by no means definitive, as the literature reveals (see Alderson (2004) and Roberts (2008) for questions and guidelines on ethics, and Cutcliffe and Ramcharan (2002) for considerations within the 'ethics-as-process' approach).

In thinking about the above principles and to provide an example for Principle 1, Geeta highlights the benefits of creating a detailed 'research information pack'. This pack was written for various audiences affected by Geeta's Ph.D. study (school-based staff, parents/carers and participants). It formed part of her ethics submission and outlined the aims of the study and the processes involved at each stage (e.g. time commitments, transcription procedures and ownership of data, confidentiality, anonymity, reporting of the findings, withdrawal, complaints procedures, and so on). Most importantly, dialogic opportunities were created for participants to engage in discussions about their involvement. At the 'pre-consent stage', Geeta's timeline provided space for participants critically to question information in the pack (see questions raised in Kellet (2010: 23)). In this way, participants were able to understand what was involved so that they could make an 'informed' decision (at that particular moment in the study).

Participants and school-based facilitators were present at a preliminary meeting where they were orally signposted through all aspects of the study. Participants were given a week's reflection time to consider their involvement after this meeting. They were encouraged to e-mail or phone the researcher as further questions arose. As a result of this 'pre-consent phase', four girls opted out. Reasons were not always given but one Hindu girl commented on her father's concern of the family aspect of the study and the breadth of the study being wider than education alone. In such cases, parents may view the researcher as a 'nosy intruder'.

Principle 1 is central in ethics – it connects to all stages of the research process and should not be seen simply as the ritual act of signed consent. If participants are to feel fully informed, they need information to be revisited and discussed, as they could feel overwhelmed early on and even 'seduced' into saying 'yes' (see Hamzeh and Oliver (2010), who outline the difficulties of negotiating informed consent and access with Muslim girls and their parents). As a 'sensitive researcher' with insights into South Asian communities and cultures, Geeta anticipated that some girls might opt out because of the heavy time commitments during A levels, parental disapproval or the personal and intrusive nature of the study. Hence, the sample size was slightly increased to account for further withdrawals at later stages. As a 'sensitive researcher', Geeta felt it was important to anticipate the potential psychological and emotional distress that could emerge as a result of participation. Participants should not leave a study with 'painful experiences' (Liamputtong 2007: 32), and although 'pain' was not discussed explicitly, participants were informed of the in-depth nature of the study and were told to discuss only those topics with which they felt comfortable. In this way, the element of 'choice' was discussed.

Participants and staff responded positively to the information pack and preliminary meeting (in contrast to the participants in Gillies and Robinson's study: clearly the sample was very different, as highlighted earlier). Some of the girls were studying A level sociology or psychology so they found the ethics aspect relevant and even interesting.

In relation to Principle 2, 'ground rules' for the study were discussed through the information pack at the initial meeting. Although the establishment of rules is clearly important, Geeta was conscious of not making the study appear too 'school like' or formal. For example, the benefits of making research reflections were outlined, but this stage was optional, depending on individuals' extra-curricular time commitments. It was further appreciated that the 'rules' may need to be personalised for each participant. Geeta prefers to use the phrase 'researcher–participant ethics framework' to 'rules', as this implies greater negotiation and less regimentation. Clearly, the needs of the sample are central here, and some samples may benefit from a more rigid set of rules or framework at the outset.

As the research conversations were led by the girls' agendas, they were crucial in planning (or rather suggesting) topics for discussion. As each participant received a verbatim transcript after each meeting, this, along with their reflective journal, acted as a guide for planning the next session. This participation and the heightened status of their 'understandings of realities are the focus of postmodern research' (Liamputtong 2007: 20). In a way, the girls were positioned as 'leaders' in the study and there was a strong recognition of the importance of their voices and views (see Ludhra and Chappell forthcoming).

To summarise, through a process of 'critical reflexivity' (reflexive writing in her journal, discussions with her supervisors, and research conversations with academic colleagues and participants), Geeta was continually reflecting on ethical issues throughout the study (see Ludhra and Chappell forthcoming; Ludhra forthcoming).

## Practice-based task 3.1  Time to reflect on the issues

### *Engaging with ethical dilemmas: working through critical incidents*

The following scenarios illustrate real-life, ethical dilemmas. Each scenario relates to some of the complex questions connected with being an 'insider' feminist researcher. Both Chrissie and Geeta are mothers researching the distinctive experiences of young people who mirror their home experiences. Parts of each scenario have been modified for the purposes of these practical exercises. Ultimately, this section is about the youth researcher-practitioner engaging in both theoretical and practical tasks.

In order to engage in a critical dialogue, we suggest you first explore your own responses and evaluate how your beliefs and philosophical perspectives would influence your decisions. Discuss your ideas within a group, where possible, working through the reflective questions by considering the challenges, opportunities, constraints and ethical dimensions/risks of each response (ethical risks may include physical, moral, verbal, psychological or emotional areas).

Each scenario commences with a short narrative regarding an ethical dilemma. Use this to position yourself 'in role' as the youth researcher-practitioner. It is not expected that these ethical dilemmas can be practically engaged with in one sitting. Each will take time to work through as conflicting responses may well be discussed.

## Ethical dilemma 3.1

### 'Safe' spaces for research conversations

You arrive at a large secondary school at 8.30 a.m. with your schedule for three 'research conversations'. The school facilitator has had difficulties in booking secluded rooms due to the busy timetable of events during the summer term. You are led to the first mobile classroom with a dividing screen running through the centre. You quickly ascertain that the room is not sound-proof or appropriate so politely express your concern. As there are no other rooms available, you decide to cancel the first interview and wait for the second participant in another area of the school. You are later guided to the library and taken to a sound-proof room with large windows. The room is located in a central area of the library so pupils have good visibility into it. Again, you politely express concern to the facilitating teacher but she feels that the girls will be agreeable to this location.

### Reflections and discussion of Ethical dilemma 3.1

- Consider how *you* would express your views or concerns to the teacher?
- What responsibilities do you as a youth researcher-practitioner have in organising 'safe spaces' for discussions?
- What are the opportunities, challenges and ethical issues/risks of going ahead with the interviews in the two designated spaces?

- Sketch and annotate a plan of an area within a school or other research site that would be considered a 'safe space' for in-depth interviews.
- How might the researcher's and participant's view of a 'safe' space differ and why?
- To what degree should young people be involved in planning or suggesting 'safe spaces' for research qualitative interviews?

## Ethical dilemma 3.2

### Blurring the researcher and friend roles

As you carry out your qualitative interviews a few girls demonstrate a real enthusiasm to engage with you as a researcher (and possibly as a friend/advisor). You have provided contact details (work e-mail address and personal mobile number) to all participants in the 'participant research pack'. You realise from the interviews that some of your respondents assume you have shared knowledge. One girl e-mailed you some in-depth research reflections. You are very excited by this enthusiastic response as the data are rich and you are thankful for the hours she has spent contributing to the project. However, she requests a further meeting on top of the three scheduled in the proposal. She texts you several times and suggests meeting at a local coffee shop in the holidays as that would be more convenient. She further requests assistance in drafting her personal statement for university. You are happy to be helpful but become concerned about the blurring of your roles.

### *Reflections and discussion of Ethical dilemma 3.2*

By drawing on your own assumptions about research relationships, write a personal statement and then address some of the dilemmas below. Discuss in pairs why you have come to the assumptions and answers to the questions.

- What are the challenges, opportunities and ethical considerations/risks of conducting additional interviews or meetings with the participant?
- Should you help her to draft her personal statement?
- How could you avoid 'overfamiliar' relationships or situations when writing your research information outline?
- Consider the challenges, opportunities and ethical risks of developing relationships with participants beyond the research questions.

- What are the challenges, benefits and risks of giving out your mobile number to participants?

## Ethical dilemma 3.3

### Revisiting 'old ghosts': I never thought about myself

During an early phase of your study, you used semi-structured interviews. Two of the young participants displayed emotional distress during these 'one-off' interviews so the interviews were terminated (one cried and the other simply could not continue). Some of the issues discussed resonated with personal experiences from the past. You had not in any way discussed sensitive or personal experiences with your participants; however, as you began to write up the research, you engaged in a process of critical reflection where you found yourself revisiting 'old ghosts' at times. This 'emotional baggage' was not something you had planned for at the outset of the study. As an 'insider' researching your 'own group', you now realise that you valuably bring your own history, knowledge and understanding of parallel experiences to the study.

### *Reflections and discussion of Ethical dilemma 3.3*

In a piece of reflexive writing at home or in your 'study space', record aspects of your own emotional history that might come to light and impact on your research narratives.

- Consider the challenges, opportunities and ethical implications for you as a youth researcher sharing experiences of the 'self' in dialogues with young people and in academic writing.
- If a participant or young person asks about areas of your personal life, how 'open' should you be?
- Consider the opportunities and ethical consequences/risks of your responses.

## Summary and recommended reading

In writing this chapter, we have provided opportunities for you to engage with real-life ethical dilemmas based on our own research experiences and the broader literature. Examples have been contextualised within theoretical frameworks and principles for ethically grounded research. Our aim has not been to answer ethical questions as this is not possible within the myriad research contexts and interactions. Our moral and ethical judgements as human beings will be affected by our philosophical perspectives and genuine care for the well-being and enhancement of young people's lives. Each young person will bring with them a preferred way of participating in your research, and it is up to you as the youth practitioner-researcher to open doors for accessing, understanding and co-constructing the possible 'darker' areas of their lived experiences. Some may not wish to share these experiences or engage with sensitive research. So how will you 'go deep' to access and represent their multi-layered views? (Swartz 2011). When engaging in deep qualitative research (and, in Geeta's case, in aspects of participatory research), Chrissie and Geeta have encountered complex organisational challenges and experienced unplanned 'emotional baggage' at personal levels. We have used our personal histories as opportunities to reflect critically on our 'insider' perspectives as members of the communities that we are researching and seeking to understand better.

To summarise, we urge you to see ethically challenging and sensitive work as potentially illuminating and as providing genuine child- and young person-centred representations. As youth researcher-practitioners, you can make a real impact only when you understand experiences from 'their' point of view and look at the world through 'their' lens. We encourage you to pose questions of the work you engage in with young people and consider ways in which power dynamics operate across the researcher/youth worker, participant, institutions, gatekeepers, and communities that young people inhabit in society at large. Moreover, throughout this chapter, we have demonstrated how ethical issues are woven throughout the research process; therefore, administrative stages involved at ethics committee level are simply the tip of the iceberg (Swartz 2011). Ethical concerns should be linked with issues of critical reflexivity, and in doing this the researcher will be better able to explore solutions for complex dilemmas that arise during the process.

There is a wealth of literature in the area of ethics and social research, but some books are particularly useful.

Alderson, P. (2004) 'Ethics', in S. Fraser, V. Lewis, S. Ding, M. Kellett and C. Robinson (eds) *Doing Research with Children and Young People*, London: Sage.

Alderson, P. and Morrow, V. (2004) *Ethics, Social Research and Consulting with Children and Young People* (2nd edn), Ilford: Barnardo's.

Greene, S. and Hogan, G. (eds) (2005) *Researching Children's Experiences: Approaches and Methods*, London, New Delhi: Sage.

Heath, S., Brooks, R., Cleaver, E. and Ireland, E. (2009) *Researching Young People's Lives*, London: Sage.

Liamputtong, P. (2007) *Researching the Vulnerable*, London, Thousand Oaks, CA, New Delhi: Sage.

## Notes

1   A critical engagement with these strategies and agendas is necessary to understand how they have been mapped out and to assess the future of child and youth matters within the coalition government's policy framework.

2  Interestingly, this research has been updated in relation to 'gay sex', visual representation and ethics. In the 1960s police officers photographed gay sex encounters to provide prosecution evidence. Decades later the material was used as art (see Biber and Dalton 2009). Tangentially, this suggests that research or images can be used for different purposes. This raises ethical questions for youth practitioners when thinking about data and their use out of context at a later date.

3  Gillick competency is based on a ruling in English law against Victoria Gillick that involved girls under the age of sixteen being assessed as sufficiently competent to decide on contraception without parental consent. As Barton and Douglas (1995: 125–126) say, 'a competent child is one who has sufficient understanding and intelligence to enable him or her to fully understand what is proposed and also sufficient discretion to enable him or her to make a wise choice in his or her own interest'.

# References

Aapola, S., Gonick, M. and Harris, A. (eds) (2005) *Young Femininity: Girlhood, Power and Social Change*, London, New York: Palgrave Macmillan.

Adler, P. and Adler, P. (1997) 'Parent-as-researcher: the politics of researching in the personal life', in R. Hertz (ed.) *Reflexivity and VOICE*, London: Sage.

Alderson, P. (2004) 'Ethics', in S. Fraser, V. Lewis, S. Ding, M. Kellett and C. Robinson (eds) *Doing Research with Children and Young People*, London: Sage.

Alldred, P. and Burman, E. (2005) 'Analysing children's accounts using discourse analysis', in S. Greene and G. Hogan (eds) *Researching Children's Experiences: Approaches and Methods*, London, New Delhi: Sage.

Alvesson, M. and Skoldberg, K. (2009) *Reflexive Methodology: New Vistas for Qualitative Research* (2nd edn), London, New Delhi: Sage.

Atkinson, D. (2004) 'Research and empowerment: involving people with learning difficulties in oral and life history research', *Disability and Society*, 19 (7): 691–702.

Barker, J. and Smith, F. (2001) 'Power, positionality and practicality: carrying out fieldwork with children', *Ethics, Place and Environment*, 4 (2):142–147.

Barker, J. and Weller, S. (2003a) '"Is it fun?" Developing children centred research methods', *International Journal of Sociological and Social Policy*, 23 (1/2): 33–58.

Barker, J. and Weller, S. (2003b) '"Never work with children?" The geography of methodological issues in research with children', *Qualitative Research*, 3 (2): 207–227.

Barton, C. and Douglas, G. (1995) *Law and Parenthood*, London: Butterworths.

Belenky, M.F., Clinchy, B.M., Goldberger, N.R. and Tarule, J.L. (1986) *Women's Ways of Knowing: The Development of Self, Voice and Mind*, New York: Basic Books.

Bennett, F. and Roberts, M. (2004) *From Input to Influence: Participatory Approaches to Research and Inquiry into Poverty*, York: Joseph Rowntree Foundation.

BERA (2004) *Revised Ethical Guidelines for Educational Research*, London: British Educational Research Association.

Biber, K. and Dalton, D. (2009) 'Making art from evidence: secret sex and police surveillance in the tearoom', *Crime, Media, Culture*, 5 (3): 243–267.

Breen, L.J. (2007) 'The researcher "in the middle": negotiating the insider/outsider dichotomy', *Australian Community Psychologist*, 19 (1): 163–174.

Bridges, N. (2009) 'Learning and change through a narrative Ph.D.: a personal narrative in progress', in S. Trahar (ed.) *Narrative Research on Learning: Comparative and International Perspectives*, Oxford: Symposium Books.

BSA (2004) *Statement of Ethical Practice for the British Sociological Association*, London: British Sociological Association.

Burgess, R. (1984) *In the Field: Introduction to Field Research*, London: Routledge.

Cahill, C. (2004) 'Defying gravity? Raising consciousness through collective research', *Children's Geographies*, 2 (2): 273–286.

Cairns, K. (2009) 'A future to voice? Continuing debates in feminist research with youth', *Gender and Education*, 21 (3): 321–335.

Chase, S.E. (1996) 'Personal vulnerability and interpretive authority in narrative research', in R. Josselson (ed.) *The narrative study of lives, Volume 4: Ethics and Process in the Narrative Study of Lives*, Thousand Oaks, CA: Sage.

Christensen, P. and James, A. (eds) (2008) *Research with Children: Perspectives and Practices*, London: Routledge.

Clough, P. (2002) *Narratives and Fictions in Educational Settings: Doing Qualitative Research in Educational Settings*, London, New York: Open University Press.

Connolly, P. (1998) *Racism, Gender Identities and Young Children: Social Relations in a Multi-ethnic, Inner-City Primary School*, London, New York: Routledge.

Cutcliffe, J.R. and Ramcharan, P. (2002) 'Levelling the playing field? Exploring the merits of the ethics-as-process approach for judging qualitative research proposals', *Qualitative Health Research*, 12 (7): 1000–1010.

David, M., Edwards, R. and Alldred, P. (2001) 'Children and school-based research: "informed consent" or "educated consent"?', *British Educational Research Journal*, 27 (3): 347–365.

DCSF (2007) *Aiming High for Young People: A Ten Year Strategy for Positive Activities*, Department for Children, Schools and Families: HMSO.

Ellis, C. and Bochner, A. (2000) 'Autoethnography, personal narrative, reflexivity: researcher as subject', in N.K. Denzin, and Y.S. Lincoln (eds) *Handbook of Qualitative Research* (2nd edn), London: Sage.

Etherington, K. (2009) 'Reflexivity: using our "selves" in narrative research', in S. Trahar (ed.) *Narrative Research on Learning: Comparitive and International Perspectives*. Oxford: Symposium.

Evans, R. and Jones, D. (2009) 'Metacognitive approaches to developing oracy', in R. Evans and D. Jones (eds) *Developing Speaking and Listening with Young Children*, London, New York: Routledge.

Flick, U. (2009) *An Introduction to Qualitative Research* (4th edn), London: Sage.

Gillborn, D. and Youdell, D. (2009) 'Critical perspectives on race and schooling', in J.A. Banks (ed.) *The Routledge International Companion to Multicultural Education*, New York and London: Routledge.

Gillies, V. and Robinson, Y. (2010a) 'Managing emotions in research with challenging pupils: some methodological reflections', *Ethnography and Education*, 5 (1): 97–110.

Gillies, V. and Robinson, Y. (2010b) 'Shifting the goalposts: researching pupils at risk of school exclusion', in M. Rob and R. Thomson (eds) *Critical Practice with Children and Young People*, Bristol: Policy Press; Milton Keynes: Open University Press.

Goodson, I. and Sikes, P. (2001) *Life History Research in Educational Settings*, Buckingham, Philadelphia: Open University Press.

Greene, S. and Hogan, G. (eds) (2005) *Researching Children's Experiences: Approaches and Methods*, London, New Delhi: Sage.

Gwynn, J. (2004) '"What about me? I live here too!" Raising voice and changing minds through participatory research', in F. Armstrong and M. Moore (eds) *Action Research for Inclusive Education: Changing Places, Changing Practices, Changing Minds*, London: Routledge.

Hamzeh, M.Z. and Oliver, K. (2010) 'Gaining research access into the lives of Muslim girls: researchers negotiating *Muslimness*, modesty, *inshallah*, and *haram*', *International Journal of Qualitative Studies in Education*, 23 (2): 165–180.

Heath, S., Brooks, R., Cleaver, E. and Ireland, E. (2009) *Researching Young People's Lives*, London: Sage.

Hertz, R. (ed.) (1997) *Reflexivity and VOICE*, London: Sage.

Hey, V. (2000) 'Troubling the autobiography of the question: re/thinking rapport and the politics of social class in feminist participant observation', in G. Walford and C. Hudson (eds) *Studies in Educational Ethnography*, Oxford: Oxford University Press.

Humphreys, L. (1970) *Tearoom Trade: Impersonal Sex in Public Places*, London: Aldine Transaction.

Kay, T.A. (2006) 'Daughters of Islam', *International Review for the Sociology of Sport*, 41 (3–4): 339–355.

Keddie, A. (2000) 'Research with young children: some ethical considerations', *Journal of Educational Enquiry*, 1 (2): 72–81.

Kellet, M. (2010) *Rethinking Children and Research: Attitudes in Contemporary Society*, London, New York: Continuum.

Kirby, P. (2004) *A Guide to Actively Involving Young People in Research: For Researchers, Research Commissioners, and Managers*, Hampshire: INVOLVE Support Unit.

Lewis, A. and Porter, J. (2004) 'Interviewing children and young people with learning disabilities: guidelines for researchers and multi-professional practice', *British Journal of Learning Disabilities*, 32: 191–197.

Liamputtong, P. (2007) *Researching the Vulnerable*, London, Thousand Oaks, CA, New Delhi: Sage.

Ludhra, G. (2010) 'Welcome to new GEA members', *Gender and Education Association Newsletter*, 14.

Ludhra, G. (forthcoming) 'Exploring the experiences of South-Asian adolescent girls: how well do semi-structured interviews "unveil" complex stories?', in S. Rizvi (ed.) *Multidisciplinary Approaches to Educational Research: Case-studies from Europe and the Developing World*, London: Routledge.

Ludhra, G. and Chappell, A. (forthcoming) '"You were quiet – I did all the marching": research processes involved in hearing the voices of South Asian girls', *International Journal of Adolescence and Youth*.

Ludhra, G. and Jones, D. (2009) '"Unveiling" complex identities: an exploration into the perspectives and experiences of South-Asian girls', *International Journal of Learning*, 16 (8): 615–628.

Miller, T. and Bell, L. (2002) 'Consenting to what? Issues of access, gate-keeping and "informed" consent', in M. Mauthner, M. Birch, J. Jessop and T. Miller (eds) *Ethics in Qualitative Research*, London: Sage.

Miller, J. and Glassner, B. (2004) 'The "inside" and the "outside": finding realities in interviews', in D. Silverman (ed.) *Qualitative Research: Theory, Method and Practice*, London: Sage.

Mirza, H. (2009) *Race, Gender and Educational Desire: Why Black Women Succeed and Fail*, London, New York: Routledge.

Moen, T. (2006) 'Reflections on the narrative research approach', *International Journal of Qualitative Methods*, 5 (4): 1–11.

Morrow, V. and Richards, M. (1996) 'The ethics of social research with children: an overview', *Children and Society*, 10: 90–105.

Murray, C. (2006) 'Peer led focus groups and young people', *Children and Society*, 20: 273–286.

Oakley, A. (1981) 'Interviewing women', in H. Roberts (ed.) *Doing Feminist Research*, London: Routledge & Kegan Paul.

O'Connor, P. (2004) 'The conditionality of status: experience-based reflections on the insider/outsider issue', *Australian Geographer*, 35 (2): 169–176.

Roberts, H. (2008) 'Listening to children: and hearing them', in P. Christensen and A. James (eds) *Research with Children: Perspectives and Practices*, London: Routledge.

Rogers, C. (2003) 'The mother/researcher in blurred boundaries of a reflexive research process', *Auto/Biography*, 11(1–2): 47–54.

Rogers, C. (2005) A sociology of parenting children identified with special educational needs: the private and public spaces parents inhabit, unpublished thesis, University of Essex.

Rogers, C. (2007) *Parenting and Inclusive Education: Discovering Difference, Experiencing Difficulty*, Basingstoke: Palgrave Macmillan.

Sikes, P. and Potts, A. (eds) (2008) *Researching Education from the Inside: Investigations from within*, London, New York: Routledge.

Silverman, D. (ed.) (2005) *Qualitative Research: Theory, Methods and Practice*, 2nd edn, London: Sage.

Smythe, W.E. and Murray, M.J. (2000) 'Owning the story: ethical considerations in narrative research', *Ethics and Behaviour*, 10 (4): 311–336.

Sutton, L., Smith, N., Dearden, C. and Middleton, S. (2007) *A Child's-Eye View of Social Difference*, York: Joseph Rowntree Foundation.

Swartz, S. (2011) '"Going deep" and "giving back": strategies for exceeding ethical expectations when researching amongst vulnerable youth', *Qualitative Research*, 11 (1): 47–68.

Thompson, R. and Holland, J. (2003) 'Hindsight, foresight and insight: the challenges of longitudinal qualitative research', *International Journal of Social Research Methodology*, 6 (3): 233–244.

Veale, A. (2005) 'Creative methodologies in participatory research with children', in S. Greene and G. Hogan (eds) *Researching Children's Experiences: Approaches and Methods*, London, New Delhi: Sage.

Walmsley, J. and Johnson, K. (2003) *Inclusive Research with People with Learning Disabilities: Past, Present and Futures*, London: Jessica Kingsley.

Ward, J. and Henderson, Z. (2003) 'Some practical and ethical issues encountered while conducting tracking research with young people leaving the "care" system', *International Journal of Social Research Methodology*, 6 (3): 255–259.

Weller, S. (2006) 'Tuning-in to teenagers! Using radio phone-in discussions in research with young people', *International Journal of Social Research Methodology*, 9 (4): 303–315.

Weller, S. (2007a) 'Researching teenagers' citizenship: democratisation *within* and *through* the research process', seminar paper, South Bank University, 17 September.

Weller, S. (2007b) *Teenagers' Citizenship: Experiences and Education*, London: Routledge.

Wilson, E. (2009) *School-based Research: A Guide for Education Students*, Los Angeles, London, New Delhi: Sage.

Woodhead, M. and Faulkner, D. (2008) 'Subjects, objects or participants? Dilemmas of psychological research with children', in P. Christensen and A. James (eds) *Research with Children: Perspectives and Practices*, London: Routledge.

<table>
<tr><td>4</td></tr>
</table>

# 4 Doing ethnography and using visual methods

Alexandra Allan

## Overview

For some time now both ethnography and visual methods have been widely used in research with young people. Owing to the rich, in-depth data that can be generated by these approaches, their applicability to a range of existing youth settings (e.g. youth clubs, detached youth work, community groups, formal educational settings), the fact that they build upon the existing skills, relationships and expertise of youth practitioners and young people alike, and their versatility in applied youth work, they have been readily taken up and adopted by a range of youth practitioners. In academic research these approaches have also been used in combination. Many commentators have noted the similarities in the way that these approaches have developed, particularly in traditional anthropological research practice (Pink 2004a; Banks 2001). Mead and Bateson's (1942) research is often held up as a classic example of this type of work; as an ethnographic approach that utilised film methods to explore young people's experiences of growing up in Balinese culture.

However, these methods have not always been so popular and they have not always been used together. Indeed, Mead is known for the vociferous way in which she lamented the lack of use of film methods in anthropological research. Many would also argue that it is only as society has become more visually literate that we have entered an era when it is possible for visual technologies to be used by researchers. Even today, when we have begun to talk about the combination of these two methods explicitly and fruitfully as a form of 'visual ethnography', and where there appears to have been a relative explosion of interest in this type of research practice, the two can still not be reduced simply to one practice. Both approaches continue to be used separately and considered as encompassing a wide variety of methods.

It is for these reasons that this chapter will largely treat the two approaches separately, in order to discuss both in the depth that they deserve, and in order to recognise them as independent approaches in their own rights. The chapter will begin by outlining *ethnography* – discussing how it has developed within the social sciences and how it continues to be practised in contemporary youth research. A section offering practical advice about conducting ethnographic research with young people will follow. The chapter will then outline visual research practice in much the same way. Each section will be laced with examples from research projects that have been undertaken with young people in order to illustrate the variety of ways in which these approaches have been adopted by researchers. Towards the end of the chapter, these discussions will be drawn together in a section that will specifically focus on visual ethnography and in a case study that will comprehensively outline a visual ethnographic research project.

## Ethnography

Although ethnography is a diverse practice with a number of possible definitions, it has widely been described as an approach to research that is based on 'direct observations', with the researcher becoming 'immersed in the field situation' (Spindler and Spindler 1992: 15). As Hammersley and Atkinson (1995: 1) elucidate, ethnography can be understood as:

> a particular method or set of methods. In its most characteristic form it involves the ethnographer participating, overtly or covertly, in people's daily lives for an extended period of time, watching what happens, listening to what is said, asking questions – in fact, collecting whatever data are available to throw light on the issues that are the focus of the research.

Ethnography is an approach that is believed to combine a number of different methods. Participant observation is often central to this grouping of methods, as ethnographers tend to participate in the everyday lives of a group for an extended period of time (months or even years) in order to engage with their traditions, cultures and practices, and to make their behaviour or way of life comprehensible to others outside of that group (Clifford and Marcus 1986). Qualitative interviewing is also often used in an informal and flexible manner. This can range from a relatively formal, semi-structured individual interview (such as those that are often witnessed in other forms of qualitative research practice) to unstructured conversations that occur in the field as a result of particular observations or incidents (Renold *et al.* 2008).

Documentary analysis is another approach that is commonly utilised in ethnographic research. Some authors believe that this method was traditionally used in ethnographic research that took place in societies where there had been little attempt to create documentary records of activity. However, this is a method that continues to be used in contemporary projects primarily because of the way in which the use of documents is thought to complement the data generated by participant observation, and allows an insight into the ways in which these groups have been (re)presented in texts and images. Ethnographers have tended to collect a wide variety of documents, including prospectuses, leaflets, posters, adverts, letters and diaries. (For further details about the specific use of documentary data and research see Chapter 7.) Although ethnographers have principally used qualitative research methods, some researchers have suggested that it is not an exclusively qualitative approach and does not preclude the use of quantitative methods (Prior 1997). It is for these reasons that ethnography is often referred to as a research approach or a methodology rather than a singular method.

However, ethnography is not just defined by the methods that ethnographers commonly utilise, for it is also well known for being an approach that is usually practised in 'natural' everyday life social settings that exist beyond and independently of the research itself (e.g. football matches, the street, a busy youth project or a community centre). The philosophy that underpins this methodology is often referred to as a form of naturalism; the idea that the social world can be understood in all its complex forms only when it is studied in its natural state (Matza 1969: 5). This is an understanding that draws on a number of different theoretical traditions (interactionism, phenomenology and hermeneutics), and as such it places particular emphasis upon exploring the meanings that guide people's behaviour in different groups, cultures and societies. This is an understanding that has developed in traditional anthropological practice. Such a tradition often regarded researchers as intrepid explorers, travelling to far-off shores to explore 'exotic' cultures; naturalism is thought to have made particular sense because it referred to the way in which these researchers explained these cultures to those 'back home'. Perhaps there is a comparison to be made between the exploration of exotic 'new lands and new peoples' in the nineteenth and early twentieth centuries and

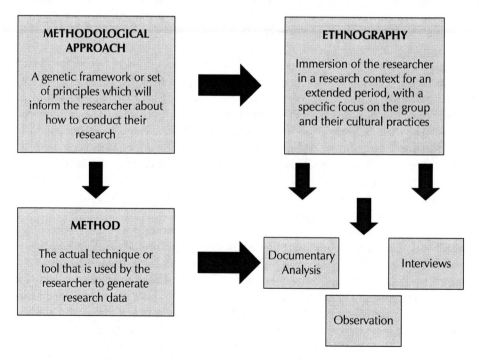

Figure 4.1 Ethnography as a research approach

contemporary ethnographies of 'exotic' youth subcultures (e.g. grungers, rude boys, hippies and Goths).

However, the concept has also been used in ethnographic research projects that have been undertaken 'closer to home'. Not all ethnographers have travelled abroad to study different social groups. As Les Back (2007: 9) describes it, this type of research is about having more of an interest in what is happening 'at the local bus stop than on some distant shore'. Indeed, Back's (1996) own research has been undertaken in the everyday settings where young people gather in South London (see below).

The Chicago School of Sociology is often thought to be the birthplace of modern sociological ethnographic research practice. This was a school that started to look at society in a new and fresh way, adopting an urban ecological approach to studying different groups in society. It was also a school where there was an insistence on 'going out and getting the seat of your pants dirty'. This approach was taken up by researchers who believed that it allowed them to get closer to their participants and gave *them* some control over the research agenda. Indeed, Agar (1986) suggests that it is the emphasis on listening to participants in ethnography that makes it so distinct. James (2001) also proposes that ethnography's insistence on listening to people is one of the reasons why it has been taken up so readily by youth researchers. Ethnography, she says, is one of the methods that has most readily allowed young people to be viewed as social actors in their own right and worthy participants (James 2001).

A great deal of ethnographic research conducted with young people has occurred in schools (perhaps because they remain the easiest contexts for researchers to access young people). However, it has not always been limited to school settings. Indeed, one of the classic ethnographic studies emanating from the Chicago School was a piece of research conducted by William Foote Whyte (1993) in the early 1940s with a group of young people in an Italian slum in Boston. With the help of one contact (Doc), who worked as his 'vouchsafe', Foote Whyte was able to spend a great deal of time on the streets with these young people, exploring their lives and experiences, the formation and structures of their gangs and their attitudes to education and work.

An example of ethnographic research undertaken with young people is provided in Box 4.1.

## Box 4.1 New ethnicities and urban culture: racisms and multiculture in young lives

Between 1985 and 1989, Les Back conducted research on two post-war council estates in South London: Riverview (predominantly a white, working-class estate) and Southgate (a multi-ethnic neighbourhood). Back's research was largely conducted within youth club settings in these two neighbourhoods, where he worked as a volunteer and in paid employment at the same time as conducting the research. Using observational methods, informal and group interviews, Back sought to explore how the young people in these neighbourhoods articulated notions of identity and ethnicity and how these were acted out within adolescent interactions.

The extract below is an example of ethnographic writing taken from Back's (1996) book about the project. The extract is used to demonstrate how the data generated in ethnographic research may be written up in order to be shared with a wider audience. This particular extract focuses on Back's observations of the interactions and play fights that occurred between the young people in these youth clubs. The extract begins with the words of the young participants and ends with Back's own analytic commentary of these events.

Tony: Yeah, come here Robert, let's 'ave a look at those hands. [Robert walks over. Steve puts his hand on the table for comparison with Robert]
Steve: Put your hand down there next to mine [Looks at Robert].
[Robert looks at Steve and puts his hand down. Steve takes the spoon out of his tea and puts it on the back of Robert's hand]
Robert: Agh – you wanker!
[Steve and Robert laugh]
Steve: What a wally.
[All three boys laugh]

There are two things I want to point out. First, the teaspoon wind-up initiates Tony into a group where 'wind-ups' are not taken as insults. Tony enters a space, or more correctly agrees to enter a space, where wind-ups are not a form of conflict. The play state is maintained. Although insults are hurled by Robert and Steve, their meanings are impotent. Secondly, although the collusion that takes place within this interaction prevents any escalation in conflict, status positions are defined. Steve and Tony establish themselves as the agents who act upon Robert – the subject – who is thereby shamed.

(Back 1996: 77)

## Criticisms, challenges and concerns

For many academics, the emphasis that ethnographers have placed on naturalism has become increasingly problematic in recent years. With the advent of post-structural theory, with the developments that have taken place within hermeneutic and feminist thinking, and with the 'crisis of representation' that is thought to have occurred within social science, many began to question whether ethnography can reflect 'reality' in any simple sense, and whether ethnographers can ever be value neutral in their practice, simply reporting on what is out there. For some, the claims that ethnographers made for 'accessing the truth' of social situations could no longer be upheld.

For many ethnographers, this has meant a move to more reflexive forms of thinking and to accounting for the inevitable role that the ethnographer plays in interpreting cultural worlds and representing them for others. This is a particularly pertinent point for youth practitioners who may be conducting research in the settings where they are already employed. Not only will these researchers have to conform to the requirements of that setting (e.g. taking on certain authoritarian roles, working to uphold existing safeguarding procedures) and establish a clear research identity for themselves (ensuring that the participants know when they are participating in the project), but they will have to acknowledge how their role as a youth worker shapes the data that they are able to generate and the analysis of their findings. As Coffey (1999: 1) argues, ethnographic fieldwork is always 'personal, emotional and identity work'.

From a post-structural perspective, others, such as Britzman (2000: 8), have described this shift in thinking as a way of 'working in the twilight of foundationalism' and a case of 'working the ruins' of ethnography. As researchers like Maclure (2002) and Youdell (2006) point out, this means re-examining our understandings of ethnography so that the 'real' that ethnography aims to explore is taken as an effect of discourses, and so that ethnography itself can be expected to summon only partial truths and fictions.

Others have attempted to describe this shift in ethnographic thinking in different ways. Les Back (2007), for example, has invited sociologists to engage with the world differently. Back argues that the capacity to hear what is going on in society has been damaged and is in need of urgent repair. What is needed, he believes, is a new form of listening: one that is multi-sensory, slow paced, open and humble. This should be a critique that is tied to the 'art of description' and captures 'life's light and heat' (Back 2007: 21). This does not simply mean listening to participants as if they were the experts of their own subjective experiences (as has commonly been the case in many traditional ethnographic studies), but rather paying attention to the insights and blindness in the accounts, having the humility and honesty to reflect on our own assumptions and interpretations as researchers, and moving constantly between theorisation and empirical detail. For Back, then, this is not simply a return to naturalism, but neither is it a rejection of ethnography simply because it cannot reflect reality in any simple sense. Adapting an analogy from Adorno, Back (2007: 21) helpfully describes this as viewing the 'truths' in ethnography as a handful of sand, where

> Most of the grains slip through our fingers, but something sticks and can be held in the palm. In a desperate attempt to hold onto these pure grains – and in the intense heat produced by the desire to know and understand – a lens is forged. It is made up equally of the grains of truth that form its elements and the hand that fashions it.

Following Back's example, many have continued to engage in ethnographic research with young people. Rather than seeing ethnography as a useless practice that cannot grasp the complexities of social life, many researchers have continued to engage with it because it allows them to get close to young people, to include their voices in research accounts and to make a difference to their lives and experiences. In recent years ethnographers have worked with many different groups of young people, focusing on a multitude of topics. Examples of this type of ethnographic research include Hodkinson's (2002) work with Goth young people, Hey's (1997) work on girls' friendship practices,

Emond's (2005) work with young people in a care home, Cullen's (2006) work on young women's smoking and drinking cultures, Cohen's (2001) work on rock cultures in Liverpool and Thornton's (1995) research on club cultures.

It is important to recognise that these examples are extremely diverse, spanning a range of approaches and utilising a number of different theoretical frameworks. Thus, as Delamont and Atkinson (1980) remind us, there is no hard and fast relationship between ethnography and any one social theory. This does not mean, however, that researchers should engage with ethnography as if it were a self-justified activity, for, as these authors suggest, ethnographers should always seek to recognise the theoretical assumptions that they bring to their research.

---

### Practice-based task 4.1  Reading task

Familiarise yourself with one of the ethnographic texts mentioned in the previous section and consider the following questions:

1   Where was the research conducted and how was it carried out?

2   How can you tell that the research is ethnographic and what do you think makes it ethnographic?

3   If you are currently engaged in work in a youth setting (e.g. youth centre, advice centre, school), what sorts of research questions would you want to address within that setting that may be supported by ethnographic research?

4   What are the problems or challenges that you may face in conducting such research?

---

## Doing ethnography

Because of the emphasis placed on being in the field and spending time with participants, it is often assumed that ethnographers can do little to prepare themselves for their research. Although ethnography involves a flexible and reflexive research design, there remain a number of principled decisions that will have to be considered before, during and after fieldwork is conducted. (See Chapter 2 for more on this.)

### Research problem

Although ethnographic research does not necessarily involve developing a hypothesis, it does require a focus on a certain issue, problem or question. This could be an issue in which the researcher has prior interest (e.g. something that they may have experienced

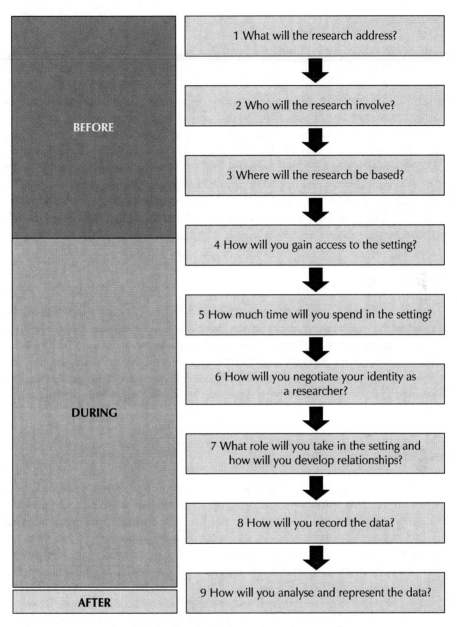

**Figure 4.2** Considerations that ethnographic researchers must address during a study

themselves). It may also be an issue that they have located in the literature (e.g. a topic that has not been addressed for some time). As Hammersley and Atkinson (1995) note, although this initial focus is vital, it is worth remembering that the focus of ethnographic research will often change across time as the participants begin to direct the researcher to matters that are important to them.

## Participants

The group with whom the ethnographer will work is also crucial to the research design. As a researcher develops their research focus they will usually have a group in mind. However, some researchers may find a group before they develop their research focus. Baym (2000), for example, spent a few months interacting with soap fans in an online discussion forum before she decided that this would become the focus of her research. Groups may also be chosen according to the personal contacts that a researcher may have or due to particular characteristics that they are seeking to represent in the study (e.g. gender, ethnicity or age). Lofland and Lofland (1995), however, suggest that one of the most fundamental questions ethnographers must ask themselves before they begin working with a group is: 'Am I reasonably able to get along with them?' The relationships that the researcher develops in the field will shape the data collection and analysis in powerful ways.

## Context/setting

The context or setting in which the research will take place is also often decided at the same time as the research problem. Researchers often limit themselves to one or two settings in which to work (e.g. one youth group or two school classes). The reason for keeping the group sizes so small and the settings to a minimum is largely due to the intensity of ethnographic research and the realisation that the more groups there are, the less time the researcher will have to spend with each. For many ethnographers, depth is considered to be far more important than breadth.

## Access and ethics

The people, the setting and the project all depend on the researcher being able to gain access to a group. This will often mean locating a 'gatekeeper' who can grant permission for this access, maybe finding someone to work as a 'vouchsafe' (to introduce you to others and to vouch for who you are and what you do), and using a range of interpersonal skills to gain the trust of the group. As with all social research, it is important that access is not viewed as a one-off event. Particularly within ethnography, access must be viewed as something that will be continually negotiated over time. Indeed, it is common for projects to expand their work and to enter new and different contexts over time. As Delamont (2002) reminds us, we must be careful not to exploit these privileges and experiences. We must remember that it is rare for researchers to gain access to all areas of social life, and as such we must afford our research participants some privacy.

## Time

Time is also an important concept in ethnography and something that often has to be negotiated at the initial point of access. In recent years there has been some concern over a rise in 'blitzkrieg' approaches to ethnography (Rist 1980; Jeffrey and Troman 2004). These have also been referred to as 'quick and dirty' modes of research. This has led a number of scholars to suggest that a period of one to two years is the ideal completion time for an ethnographic project (see, for example, Nayak's (2003) account of living on an estate with his young participants and conducting research over a three-year period). However, many researchers (and certainly students) simply do not have this amount of time to complete their projects because external funding bodies and those commissioning the research generally impose strict deadlines on them. Therefore, some researchers have begun to talk about using an 'ethnographic approach' in their work. This signals the intent to study a group in *some* detail without committing the time that a 'full-blown' ethnography may demand.

## Roles and identities

In line with Gold's (1958) work, it has conventionally been suggested that there are four roles that researchers need to choose between when they employ observational methods in their research:

1 participant as observer
2 full participant
3 observer as participant
4 full observer.

It is similarly proposed that a degree of 'impression management' needs to be maintained by ethnographers in order to fit into certain social settings – involving dressing correctly, speaking correctly and taking up pre-prepared roles within institutions (Lofland and Lofland 1995). Although many have since questioned these roles and strategies for self-management (asking whether anyone could ever be a full participant in a group, whether it is useful to distinguish between the researcher as an insider or outsider to the group, and whether they will only ever be seen in such static ways (Coffey 1999)), many ethnographers do still acknowledge that researchers have to make certain practical decisions relating to their role and identity – including from where they choose to observe and how involved they are with a group.

## Relationships

The same practical considerations are often not made in advance in terms of research relationships, as these will usually be negotiated at the time. However, ethnographers are often advised to consider what form these relationships may take and how they may react should certain behaviour arise. For example, how would a youth researcher react to illegal or unruly behaviour or to sexual advances? Another crucial consideration for youth researchers is how power will play out in their relationships with young people and how they may deal with a potential imbalance of power between them as adult researchers or practitioners and their young participants. Many researchers recognise that there is no simple way to deal with these issues; that it is not just about researchers somehow concealing their 'adult' characteristics or acting as if they were young people themselves. As Christensen (2004) reminds us, it is not simply a matter of adults having power over vulnerable young people in research. Power is continuously produced and negotiated throughout the research process and this means that researchers will need to be reflexive about the range of different relationships, roles and identities that they engage in during the process.

## Recording data

One of the main ways in which data is recorded during ethnographic research is through field notes, which are taken by the researcher to record what they observe and what people say to them. The advice that is commonly given to ethnographic researchers is that it is always best for these notes to be written as soon as possible and to avoid relying too heavily on memory. For some researchers, this will mean jotting down notes as they observe; for others, it will mean taking extensive notes as soon as they get home at the end of the day. Researchers are also often advised to take time over these notes in order to develop them as fully as possible. Perhaps one of the most difficult tasks for any ethnographer is to know what to note down when they first begin to observe. Spradley (1980) offers a useful checklist, including:

- spaces
- actors
- activity
- events
- times
- goals
- feelings.

In addition, Gordon *et al.* (2005) advise researchers to focus on inactivity and silence as well as action, for they believe this broadens the observational field and allows for more attention to be paid to issues of space and embodiment.

---

## Box 4.2  Field note example

The following example of a field note is taken from Marnina Gonick's (2003) ethnographic research with young women in one school in Toronto. In this extract she concentrates on providing a description of the context in which her research was based:

---

It is March 1, 1995, three months before the end of the school year which would also mark the end of two and a half years I have spent in the school. The hall is full of boisterous students, just released from their desks by the ringing of the bell signalling the lunch break. The bench I am leaning against is my waiting place. Here, the girls that I have been working with on a video project assemble to ascend the two flights of stairs together, to our meeting room. The school foyer is brightly painted in non-institutional purples and blues and decorated with student artwork: paintings with seasonal themes, the award-winning posters in the school-wide competition in celebration of Anti-Racism Day, and the elaborate cloth murals from some long ago project, hanging permanently from the ceiling.

(Gonick 2003: 6)

## *Analysis and representation*

The methods of analysis and forms of representation that an ethnographer chooses will often depend upon the theoretical framework underpinning the project. (For a full account of these different approaches, see Hammersley and Atkinson (1995) and Coffey and Atkinson (1996).) Like all research projects, ethnographic studies reach a stage where the researcher must leave the field and a formal process of analysis must begin. However, in line with qualitative principles, many ethnographers will view analysis as an ongoing and cyclical process that takes place alongside the collection and generation of data. This will often involve making initial analytic memos in field notes, asking participants to confirm or review initial hunches and ideas, and taking time to read the data in order to direct future fieldwork.

Having outlined ethnography and its use in youth research, the next section will establish what visual research is and how it may be undertaken by youth researchers.

## Visual methods

The term 'visual research' is often used to describe projects where researchers make use of visual materials (such as film, photography or drawing) in the research process, either to generate data or as a form of data itself. Many commentators have noted the centrality of visual images in contemporary social life (Rose 2004; Berger 1972). Some have also linked this to research practice, suggesting that we have witnessed a 'visual turn' in the social sciences, meaning that visual methods have become increasingly accepted as a valid tool for conducting research (Thomson 2008). Yet, despite these claims relating to the contemporary nature of this 'occularcentrism', visual methods cannot be regarded as a particularly recent phenomenon. In common with ethnography, they are thought to have strong roots in traditional anthropological practice. Early anthropologists, such as Mead and Bateson (1942), for example, were reported to have been particularly keen on using film methods to observe the cultures and practices of other societies. Mead (1995) was certainly strongly in favour of setting up the film camera and leaving it to run in a relatively unobtrusive manner in order to capture as much action as possible.

Pink (2004a) believes that some other disciplines, like sociology, did not 'catch on' to the use of these practices for some time after anthropology had adopted them. Early studies are noted for viewing and using images in particular ways – within the positivist research tradition and in a 'realist' sense. During this period, images were very much seen as reflections of the social world. It was felt that these images could capture the 'facts' of the social world and that researchers could interpret their contents in simple ways in order to illuminate the understanding of social behaviours. Collier's (1967) book was particularly influential at this time, as he claimed that visual methods could be used as a systematic way to observe the social world. Collier made the distinction between the 'fiction' that he felt was contained in traditional films and the 'facts' that were the object of serious visual research.

Yet, as other forms of research practice and representation began to be questioned during the so-called 'crisis of representation' in the social sciences, so did this understanding of visual research. As Thomson (2008) suggests, many researchers began to question the idea that an image could be viewed as a simple 'window on the world'. Just as they began to see words as human constructions, researchers also began to see images as constructed and culturally specific. Rather than being understood as neutral, many researchers came to recognise that images were constructed through the processes of selection (e.g. what is included in the image), manipulation (e.g. editing) and display (e.g. how it is exhibited). Pink (2004a) refers to this as a newly 'reflexive' form of visual research, and Rose (2004) summarises the main viewpoints that researchers working from this understanding share:

1    Images should be treated seriously in research.
2    The social conditions and effects of visual objects need to be considered.
3    Researchers need to account for their own particular ways of looking at images.

Visual research is often discussed in relation to the researcher's role in the collection or generation of images in a research project. For example, Banks (2001) has famously made the distinction between visual research where the researcher creates the images, visual research where the researcher discusses ready-made images, and research where the researcher and participants collaborate to generate new images. However, visual research is also categorised according to the technology that is used to create the data or the form that the images take.

## Photography

Researchers have often used photography because cameras are readily available (especially with the advances that have been made in relation to digital and mobile phone cameras in recent years) and because people are often very familiar with photographic practice. Many of the well-known researchers of our time have engaged in photographic research. Pierre Bourdieu's (1990) work on class practices and photography is just one example. Indeed, Pink (2004a) comments that the camera has long been seen as a mandatory tool for some researchers.

Researchers will not always create new images during the research process. Rather, they will sometimes use images that already exist. These may take the form of a photo elicitation interview, where the researcher will ask the participants to discuss images in order to generate information. This could involve using old family photographs and certain forms of 'memory work' in order to elicit biographical information from participants.

Under the influence of Harper (2002), however, many researchers now prefer to refer to these interviews as 'photo feedback sessions'. This new term recognises that interviews do not simply elicit responses from participants, but instead involve negotiations between the researcher and the participant, who work together to construct meanings around the images. As Okely (1994: 51) notes, in her project it was a case of her and the participants 'piecing together the memories' and 'working together [to] create a synthesised whole' from images that were found in each participant's collection.

Other researchers may prefer to generate new images within a research project, either themselves or by giving a camera to their participants. In Pink's (2004a) account of Spanish bullfighting culture, she discusses the way in which she took photographs of bullfights as a way of observing and entering the culture. As the project progressed, Pink was invited to take photographs at particular events, meaning that she was able to learn a great deal about the importance of images and the ways in which this group sought to represent these practices. Mizen (2005), on the other hand, gave disposable cameras to the young people that he worked with so that they could take photographs of the employment practices in which they were engaged. Some researchers have also used this type of participant-led photography as a form of action research, sometimes referred to as 'photo voice' – a method that aims to use photographs to access the voices of marginalised groups so that they can be used to change their lives for the better (Wang and Burris 1997; Mitchell *et al.* 2006).

## *Film*

Researchers have also used camcorders to produce films that capture their participants' experiences. As technology has progressed, this practice has become cheaper and more viable for researchers. Indeed, we now live in an era where websites like YouTube have made it incredibly easy for people to share moving images with one another, where musical devices like iPods have reasonable recording facilities built into them, and where various forms of editing software can be downloaded for free usage. Scholars like Heath *et al.* (2009) suggest that it is for these very reasons (their relative cheapness and the fact that they can be shared and manipulated easily) that video methods have become increasingly common in research practice in recent years.

Some researchers may use film methods as a simple form of documentation. It is common to find camcorders being used as additional recording devices during observations or interviews. This could be because they add another level of 'vision' to the research project – allowing the researcher to focus on one aspect with the knowledge that the camera will pick up other forms of action. It may also be because it allows the researcher to have a permanent record of events that can be viewed on multiple occasions. However, it is important that researchers approach this practice with some caution – not viewing it as either simple or neutral – for it will depend on a number of decisions (e.g. where the camera is placed and what it focuses on) and it will often generate an inordinate amount of data that could be difficult to transcribe and analyse.

Other researchers have generated their own films by using the camcorder in more creative ways. This can take the form of video tours (see, for example, Pink's (2004b) work on domestic cleaning practices), 'guerrilla-style' roving films (a mobile filming method that follows participants around to see the world from their perspective) or even observational films (attempts to film for lengthy periods without scripts or direction from the researcher; see http://www.visualanthropology.net for examples). As camcorders have become cheaper, researchers have also engaged their participants in more collaborative film projects. Examples include Holliday's (2000) use of camcorders to ask participants to make video diaries, Renold *et al.*'s (2008) attempts to engage young people in work with a professional film-maker, and Noyes' (2008) use of a camcorder in a *Big Brother*-style diary room where young people were asked to record their thoughts and feelings about their approaches to learning mathematics.

## Drawing/mapping/artwork

Researchers have also used multiple forms of artwork and creative methods to generate visual research data or to examine existing images. Pink (2004a) suggests that there is a long history in the use of drawing in research, and Rose (2004) indicates that social geographers have used mapping techniques for a number of years (e.g. participants are asked to draw maps or diagrams of the spaces that they inhabit). Within media and cultural studies, certain forms of creative drawing and collage have also been used. For example, in their study of the media representation of sexual relationships, Buckingham and Bragg (2008) asked young people to create scrapbooks containing images, notes and jottings that they collected from a variety of different media sources in order to represent their own views on these issues. Of course, such approaches are very similar to those that practitioners may already be undertaking in youth work settings (e.g. collages, artwork, mind maps), demonstrating their applicability in research with young people.

In recent years there has been an astounding take-up of visual research methods in projects that involve young people. This is often claimed to be due to the reduced cost of equipment and young people's developing visual literacies. Examples of visual research projects undertaken with young people include Bloustien's (2003) film work with young women who created and edited their own film about their everyday experiences, Young and Barrett's (2000) use of multiple visual methods (photography, drawing and mapping) with Brazilian street children, Allen's (2009) photographic work on sexuality and sexual identity, and Gonick's (2003) work with young girls to write scripts and develop a film as a way of exploring subjectivity formation.

A major reason why visual research methods have been so popular in youth research is due to the belief that they can be easily implemented in a collaborative format (Banks 2001). Not only are visual research methods often described as fun and creative practices that young people will enjoy; they are often thought to offer researchers access to voices of different groups of young people (e.g. those who have difficulty with words (see Thomson 2008)). However, a number of academics have questioned this growing trend and have suggested that these collaborative visual practices need to be subject to closer scrutiny. Buckingham and De Block (2007), for example, argue that we cannot simply assume that all children know how to use digital technology, that they always find it fun to use and that it can be taken up in simple ways to produce visual statements that easily illuminate their everyday lives.

In a similar manner, Piper and Frankham (2007) call for greater attention to be paid to the ways in which young people's photographs are used and interpreted in participatory projects. They suggest that photographs do not speak for themselves in any simple way, that their meanings are not transparently available to audiences through some sort of direct connection with the artist's mind, but that they are often interpreted by adult researchers who bring their own 'iconoclastic' baggage to the process. As such, Piper and Frankham believe that researchers need to take more responsibility in their interpretation and representation of these images; that they need to 'unlearn their own privilege', to consider alternative explanations, to think about what is not being said and cannot be spoken, and to challenge the 'transparency of the gaze'.

## Doing visual research

The variety of examples given in the previous sections illustrate that there is no one way in which to approach visual research and that there can be no 'blueprints' or simple recipes for success. However, we argue that these approaches have considerable promise for youth research and for researcher-practitioners researching young people's worlds. However, we need to flag up a number of key considerations.

### Ethics

Visual research does not necessarily entail an entirely different set of ethical guidelines or practice from other forms of social research. There are, however, some aspects of the research practice that come to the foreground more readily in visual research than in other projects. One key aspect is anonymity, for research participants cannot always be assured full anonymity if images of them are to be included in the reports, articles or presentations that arise from the research project. Although some authors may question the anonymity that written texts offer participants (given the level of detail that is used), there is certainly something more immediate about visual images that means that faces and places can be recognised more readily.

This has caused particular concern for researchers working with young people, for they are often working in contexts where there are already limits imposed on how young people are visually represented and in a climate of fear (see Allan and Cullen 2008). No one solution has been offered to address these concerns. Some researchers will choose not to share images as they disseminate their research (viewing them more as part of the research process than as data that need to be seen). Others will use images in some forms of dissemination practice (e.g. in presentations where the images cannot be taken away by members of the audience). Still others will choose to pixellate faces or trace the images so that the participants are not easily identifiable.

Visual researchers are also often concerned about issues of ownership, permission and informed consent. Some useful information on these issues can be gleaned from the professional codes of ethical conduct in visual research that have been created by such research organisations as the British Sociological Association (see http://www.britsoc. co.uk/equality/Statement+Ethical+Practice.html). However, as Pink (2004a) suggests, these are only guidelines, and in many cases these issues will have to be worked out on an individual project basis.

## Technology

Decisions relating to technology will often depend on economic factors. However, they may also rest upon the nature of the project and the role of the researcher within the project. Pink (2004a) believes that the technology used in a project will become part of the researcher's identity within the field, which is one of the reasons why she suggests it is essential for researchers to consider its usage in detail. Pink also suggests that gaining good knowledge of the existing visual culture of a group is important before fieldwork begins. This could involve running a pilot study to find out what equipment the group normally use, how groups view visual images and how they are constructed and shared. Publications such as those produced by Heath *et al.* (2009) provide detailed checklists to help researchers assess the technology that they will use. For example, will the camcorder have to be transported? Do you need a colour LCD screen? Will you need an external microphone?

## Analysis

Visual researchers will utilise numerous methods of analysis. A good account of these different methods can be found in Rose's (2004) book, which discusses three different ways of analysing images:

1    in terms of their production (looking at the context in which images are produced);
2    in terms of the image itself (looking at the content);
3    in relation to the audience (in terms of the meanings that are given to them by different groups of people).

Analysis, then, is very much tied to the theoretical framework that underpins any research. Therefore, decisions about analysis of visual images can often not be left until the data have been generated.

The next section will conclude the chapter by drawing ethnography and visual research together in order to address how they have been used in combination as a form of 'visual ethnography'.

## Visual ethnography

In recent years visual methods have become increasingly incorporated into the research practices of ethnographic researchers, so much so that it is not uncommon now for researchers to define themselves as 'visual ethnographers'. Although many have argued that there is nothing particularly distinct about the images that are used in ethnographic research, there is recognition that ethnography and visual methods have a great deal to offer one another:

> Ethnographic research is . . . intertwined with visual images and metaphors. When ethnographers produce photographs or videos, these visual texts, as well as the experience of producing and discussing them, become part of their ethnographic knowledge . . . In ethnography images are as inevitable as sounds, smells, textures and tastes, words or any other aspect of culture or society. Although ethnographers should not be obliged to make the visual central to their work, they might explore its relation to other senses and discourses.
>
> (Pink 2004a: 21)

In order to focus on what visual ethnography might look like in practice, Case study 4.1 outlines one project where these two approaches to research were combined and where visual ethnographic data were produced.

---

### Case study 4.1

### An ethnographic exploration of the construction of gendered subjectivities in elite educational institutions (Allan 2010)

---

### Overview

This case study refers to two research projects undertaken by the author of this chapter. The first project was based in one single-sex, private primary school and took place with a class of twenty-five young girls (aged ten and eleven). The second project was based in two private secondary schools with young people aged sixteen and seventeen. One of these schools was single-sex and the other had recently become co-educational. Although the two projects can be viewed as independent of each another (they focused on slightly different concerns and were separated by a period of four years), they are also connected in a number of ways (both had a focus on the construction of young femininities in elite education – on what it meant to be a young woman in this setting – and worked with some of the same young people as part of a longitudinal follow-up study).

## Methods

In the first project visual methods were primarily used in a marginal capacity. But as the research developed photographic methods came to play a particularly large role in the project because of the ways in which they were understood to complement the study of identity constitution. As Holliday (2000: 516) suggests, visual methods can be understood as a 'particularly post-modern medium' that can be used to 'capture the ways in which different subjects may be situated in specific configurations of discourse whilst making those discourses open for examination as they recur in different images'.

Alongside participant observation, focus group interviews and individual interviews, the girls participating in the project were asked to create photographic diaries that represented their gendered identities (what it meant to them to be a girl). The girls were each given a photography pack to use as part of the project, including a disposable camera, a pack of photographic activities, a notebook and a diary.

At the same time as the girls were creating their photographic diaries, they were also invited to join a lunchtime photography club where they further explored what it meant to construct a photograph. The club was not aimed at introducing the girls to techniques for taking good photographs (the researcher had no particular photographic expertise, and nor was it something that this group needed). Rather, the sessions were aimed at looking at photographs critically in order to examine the meanings that the girls invested in their own images and the discourses that they drew on in their own presentation of self. The club culminated in a one-day photography workshop where the girls collaborated with a professional photographer to produce a range of portrait prints. All of the images created by the girls were discussed in photo feedback interviews with the researcher and analysed alongside the other research data generated in the project (see Allan 2004, 2008).

In the second project the young women were given the opportunity to choose how they wanted to be involved in the project. Many of them had worked with the researcher previously and were keen to use visual methods again, so film-making became a central part of the research process. The young people began this work by bringing in a set of photographs to discuss with the researcher in a photo feedback interview. These were often a combination of images that they had either taken on one of the project's digital cameras or had brought in from their own personal collections, but they all represented their experiences of life in a private sixth-form college and their identities as young men and women.

After the interviews, some of the young people worked on creating 'photomatics' – short films made from combinations of these still images. As the project progressed, the young people also began to work together to develop a script and a storyboard for a film that would represent their experiences. At the end of the project they worked with a professional film-maker to produce and edit the film so that it could be shown to a group of their friends and family in their own dissemination event at a local arts centre (see Allan 2010).

## Conclusions

The use of photographic methods in these projects was exciting and methodologically rich. The visual methods appeared to have a particular resonance with their own school culture. The activities used in conjunction with these visual methods also generated a vast amount of data, including: in-depth field notes of all sessions, stories, monologues and written extracts about other photographers' work, interview transcripts from the photographic feedback sessions, scribblings, drawings and notes collected in the notebooks, and illustrations and captions used in the photographic diaries. Although the images and films themselves have been used in various dissemination activities, it was the process of producing these images that we deemed particularly useful in generating the richest ethnographic data and which allowed for a more complex picture of these young people's identities to emerge.

## Practice-based task 4.2 Analysing visual images

Look at Image 4.1 and try to answer the following questions:

1 What do you think you can tell about this image from the content contained within it?

2 What do your interpretations tell you about your own viewing practice and the meanings that you bring with you to this image?

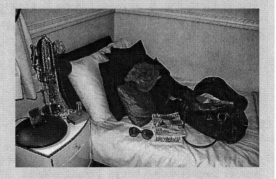

Image 4.1 Bedroom culture

3　What else would you like to know about the context in which this image was created?

4　How would you design a visual ethnographic project that sought to explore young people's 'bedroom cultures'?

5　Which technologies/methods and practices would you employ and why?

6　Can you consider what ethical issues you may need to engage with in a youth practice setting?

## Summary of main points

- Both visual methods and ethnography have a long tradition of being utilised in youth research, owing to the in-depth data that they generate, the way in which they build upon the existing skills, roles and relationships of youth practitioners and young people, and because of their versatility in applied youth work.
- Ethnography can be understood as a research approach involving practitioner-researchers immersing themselves in a social setting to observe and participate in the lives and cultural practices of a particular group. It involves the use of a number of different methods, including participant observation, interviews and documentary analysis.
- There are several principled decisions that an ethnographic researcher will have to make before, during and after they conduct their research. Some major considerations for youth practitioners may include establishing an identity as a researcher, acting within existing youth work regulations and acknowledging how their role shapes their interpretations of the data.
- Visual research is a term used to describe projects that utilise or produce visual material (e.g. films, photographs, drawing, artwork). Visual research has become widely practised in youth work settings because of the recent reductions in the cost of equipment and the way in which it builds on young people's developing visual literacies, and because it can be used in a collaborative fashion. Visual ethnography involves incorporating visual techniques in ethnographic practice (e.g. producing or analysing images alongside the use of other methods).

## Further reading

All of these texts provide a good overview of issues raised in this chapter.

Bloustien, G. (2003) *Girl Making: A Cross-cultural Ethnography on the Processes of Growing up Female*, Oxford: Berghan Books.

Coffey, A., Atkinson, P., Delamont, S., Lofland, L. and Lofland, J. (eds) (2001) *Handbook of Ethnography*, London: Sage.

Hammersley, M. and Atkinson, P. (1995) *Ethnography: Principles in Practice*, London: Routledge.

Pink, S. (2004a) *Doing Visual Ethnography*, London: Sage.

Pink, S. (2007) *Visualising Ethnography*. http://www.lboro.ac.uk/departments/ss/visualising_ethnography/ (accessed 28 April 2011).

# References

Agar, M. (1986) *Speaking of Ethnography*, Thousand Oaks, CA: Sage.

Allan, A. (2004) 'Using photographic diaries to research the gender and academic identities of young girls', in G. Walford, B. Jeffreys and G. Troman (eds) *Methodological Issues and Practices in Ethnography*, London: Elsevier.

Allan, A. (2008) 'Snapshots of subjectivities: using photographic methods in identity research with young people', paper presented at the Childhood and Youth Conference, Sheffield University, July.

Allan, A. (2010) 'Power, participation and privilege: methodological lessons from research with elite young people', paper presented at the Youth 2010 Conference, Surrey University, July.

Allan, A. and Cullen, F. (2008) 'Picturing innocence, innocent pictures? Representation and the use of self-directed photography in studies of children and young people's cultural worlds', paper presented at the Using Visual Methods in Research Examining Children's Cultural Worlds Seminar, Cardiff University, April.

Allen, L. (2009) '"Snapped": researching the sexual cultures of schools using visual methods', *Qualitative Studies in Education*, 22 (5): 54–61.

Back, L. (1996) *New Ethnicities and Urban Culture: Racisms and Multiculture in Young Lives*, London: Routledge.

Back, L. (2007) *The Art of Listening*, Oxford: Berg.

Banks, M. (2001) *Visual Methods in Social Research*, London: Sage.

Baym, N. (2000) *Tune in, Log on: Soaps, Fandom and Online Community*, Thousand Oaks, CA: Sage.

Becker, H. (1995) 'Visual sociology, documentary photography or photojournalism (almost) all a matter of context', *Visual Sociology*, 10 (1–2): 5–14.

Berger, J. (1972) *Ways of Seeing*, London: Penguin.

Bloustien, G. (2003) *Girl Making: A Cross-cultural Ethnography on the Processes of Growing up Female*, Oxford: Berghan Books.

Bourdieu, P. (ed.) (1990) *Photography: A Middle-brow Art*, Cambridge: Polity.

British Sociological Association (2002) *Statement of Ethical Practice*. http://www.britsoc.co.uk/equality/63.htm (accessed 30 July 2010).

Britzman, D.P. (2000) 'Post structural ethnography', in E. St Pierre and W.S. Pillow (eds) *Working the Ruins: Feminist Post-structural Theory and Methods in Education*, London: Routledge.

Buckingham, D. and Bragg, S. (2008) 'Scrapbooks as a resource in media research with young people', in P. Thomson (ed.) *Doing Visual Research With Children and Young People*, London: Routledge.

Buckingham, D. and De Block, L. (2007) *Global Children, Global Media: Migration, Media and Childhood*, Basingstoke: Palgrave.

Christensen, P. (2004) 'Children's participation in ethnographic research: issues of power and representation', *Children and Society*, 18: 165–76.

Clifford, J. and Marcus, G.E. (eds) (1986) *Writing Culture: The Poetics and Politics of Ethnography*, Berkeley: University of California Press.

Coffey, A. (1999) *The Ethnographic Self: Fieldwork and the Representation of Identity*, London: Sage.

Coffey, A. and Atkinson, P. (1996) *Making Sense of Qualitative Data: Complementary Research Strategies*, London: Sage.

Cohen, S. (2001) *Rock Culture in Liverpool: Popular Music in the Making*, Oxford: Oxford University Press.

Collier, J. (1967) *Visual Anthropology: Photography as Research Method*, Albuquerque: University of New Mexico Press.

Cullen, F (2006) '"Two's up and poncing fags": young women's smoking practices and gift exchange', paper presented at Girls and Education 3–16 ESRC seminar series, Lancaster University, 7 June.

Cullen, F. (2010) 'I was kinda paralytic: pleasure, peril and teenage girls' drinking cultures', in C. Jackson, C. Paechter and E. Renold (eds) *Girls and Education 3–16*, Buckingham: Open University Press.

Delamont, S. (2002) *Fieldwork in Educational Settings: Methods, Pitfalls and Perspectives*, London: Routledge.

Delamont, S. and Atkinson, P. (1980) 'The two traditions in educational ethnography', *British Journal of the Sociology of Education*, 1 (2): 139–52.

Emond, R. (2005) 'Ethnographic methods with children and young people', in S. Greene and D. Hogan (eds) *Researching Children's Experience*, London: Sage.

Foote Whyte, W. (1993) *Street Corner Society: The Social Structure of an Italian Slum*, Chicago: University of Chicago Press.

Gold, R.L. (1958) 'Roles in sociological field observation', *Social Forces*, 36: 217–33.

Gonick, M. (2003) *Between Femininities: Ambivalence, Identity and the Education of Girls*, New York: State University New York Press.

Gordon, T., Holland, J., Lahelma, E. and Tolonen, T. (2005) 'Gazing with intent: ethnographic practice in classrooms', *Qualitative Research*, 5 (1): 113–31.

Hammersley, M. and Atkinson, P. (1995) *Ethnography: Principles in Practice*, London: Routledge.

Harper, D. (2002) 'Talking about pictures: a case for photo-elicitation', *Visual Studies* 17 (1): 13–26.

Heath, C., Hindmarsh, J. and Luff, P. (2009) *Video in Qualitative Research: Analysing Social Interaction in Everyday Life*, London: Sage.

Hey, V. (1997) *The Company She Keeps*, Buckingham: Open University Press.

Hodkinson, P. (2002) *Goth: Identity, Style and Subculture*, Oxford: Berg.

Holliday, R. (2000) 'We've been framed: visualising methodology', *Sociological Review*, 48 (4): 503–21.

James, A. (2001) 'Ethnography and childhood', in A. Coffey, P. Atkinson, S. Delamont, L. Lofland and J. Lofland (eds) *Handbook of Ethnography*, London: Sage.

Jeffrey, B. and Troman, G. (2004) 'Time for ethnography', *British Educational Research Journal*, 30 (4): 535–48.

Lofland, L. and Lofland, J. (1995) *Analyzing Social Settings: A Guide to Qualitative Observation and Analysis*, London: Wadsworth.

Maclure, M. (2002) *Discourse in Educational and Social Research*, Buckingham: Open University Press.

Matza, D. (1969) *Becoming Deviant*, Englewood Cliffs, NJ: Prentice-Hall.

Mead, M. (1995) 'Visual anthropology in a discipline of words', in P. Hockings (ed.) *Principles of Visual Anthropology*, The Hague: Mouton.

Mead, M. and Bateson, G. (1942) *Balinese Character: A Photographic Analysis*, New York: New York Academy of Sciences.

Mitchell, C., Stuart, J., Rehobile, M. and Nkwanyana, C.B. (2006) '"Why we don't go to school on Fridays": on youth participation through photo voice in rural KwaZulu-Natal', *McGill Journal of Education*, 41 (3): 1–17.

Mizen, P. (2005) 'A little light work? Children's images of their labour', *Visual Studies*, 20 (2): 124–39.

Nayak, A. (2003) *Race, Place and Globalisation: Youth Cultures in a Changing World*, Oxford: Berg.

Neale, B. and Flowerdew, J. (2003) 'Time, texture and childhood: the contours of longitudinal qualitative research', *International Journal of Social Research Methods* 6 (3): 189–99.

Noyes, A. (2008) 'Using video diaries to investigate learner trajectories', in P. Thomson (ed.) *Doing Visual Research with Children and Young People*, London: Routledge.

Okely, J. (1994) 'Vicarious and sensory knowledge of chronology and change: ageing in rural France', in K. Hastrup and P. Hervik (eds) *Social Experience and Anthropological Knowledge*, London: Routledge.

Pink, S. (2004a) *Doing Visual Ethnography*, London: Sage.

Pink, S. (2004b) *Home Truths: Gender, Domestic Objects and Everyday Life*, Oxford: Berg.

Piper, H. and Frankham, J. (2007) 'Seeing voices and hearing pictures: image as discourse and the framing of image-based research', *Discourse: Studies in the Cultural Politics of Education*, 28 (3): 373–87.

Prior, L. (1997) 'Following in Foucault's footsteps: text and content in qualitative research', in D. Silverman (ed.) *Qualitative Research: Theory, Method and Practice*, London: Sage.

Renold, E., Holland, S., Ross, N. and Hillman, A. (2008) 'Becoming participant: problematising informed consent in participatory research with young people in care', *Qualitative Social Work*, 7 (4): 431–51.

Rist, R.C. (1980) 'Blitzkreig ethnography: on the transformation of a method into movement', *Educational Researcher*, 9 (2): 8–10.

Rose, G. (2004) *Visual Methodologies: An Introduction to the Interpretation of Visual Materials*, London: Sage.

Spindler, G. and Spindler, L. (1992) 'Cultural process and ethnography: an anthropological perspective', in M.D. Lecompte, W.L. Milroy and J. Priessle (eds) *The Handbook of Qualitative Research in Education*, New York: Academic Press.

Spradley, J.P. (1980) *Participant Observation*, New York: Holt, Rhinehart and Winston.

Taylor, S. (2001) *Ethnographic Research: A Reader*, London: Sage.

Thomson, P. (ed.) (2008) *Doing Visual Research with Children and Young People*, London: Routledge.

Thornton, S. (1995) *Club Cultures: Music, Media and Subcultural Capital*. Cambridge: Polity Press.

Wang, C. and Burris, M.A. (1997) 'Photovoice: concept, methodology, and use for participatory needs assessment', *Health Education and Behaviour*, 24: 369–87.

Youdell, D. (2006) *Impossible Bodies, Impossible Selves: Exclusions and Student Subjectivities*, London: Springer.

Young, L. and Barrett, H. (2000) 'Adapting visual methods: action research with Kampala street children', *Area*, 33 (2): 141–52.

<table>
| 5 | # Asking questions |
</table>

# 5 Asking questions

## Interviews and evaluations

### Clare Choak

## Overview

This chapter provides an introduction to approaches that researcher-practitioners might take when using interviews and evaluations. The chapter covers different types of interview, developing and designing questions, and the coding and analysis of data. It will also consider the current significance of evaluation studies in practice.

In youth research, interviews are most frequently used to explore the lives and viewpoints of young people as they can facilitate in-depth responses to complex research questions. Youth work (and similar practices) is fundamentally based on communication – therefore, asking questions and listening to others is a skill which successful workers are likely to possess already. Additionally, collecting information about young people's lives and evaluating it in relation to their individual biography and organisational profile is part of being a youth practitioner. Evaluation research is increasingly important to youth practitioners, with its growing significance in youth and educational practice settings in developing and shaping policy and practice. Whilst quantitative research currently remains the most common form of monitoring and evaluation in many practice settings, qualitative research is just as important in order to support, supplement or contradict existing quantitative research findings and explore the lives of individuals and groups in greater depth.

Qualitative research is the most appropriate choice for collecting data which contextualises the feelings, meanings and experiences of individuals and groups. It tends to be adopted by those who value 'people's knowledge, values and experiences as meaningful and worthy of exploration' (Bryne 2004: 182). Finding out about the lives and opinions of young people involves exploring many aspects of who they are. Choosing an approach for your study depends upon which one will provide you with the most appropriate version of social 'reality'. Qualitative research allows for exploration and new discoveries through 'belief in a constructed reality' (Bergman 2008: 13), and it is underpinned by the notion that reality can be constructed through the eyes of participant and interviewer. Its focus, then, is the interpretation of relations within a social context and the impact of power relations between researcher and the researched.

Whilst it is important to acknowledge differences between yourself and your interviewees, youth practitioners will already have established ways of building rapport and talking to their clients. Interviewing and understanding young people should make youth research more straightforward for youth workers than it is for those who do not work with young people on a regular basis, although various professional assumptions can obscure some aspects of young people's lives and circumstances.

## Qualitative interviewing

We are living in what has been referred to as an 'interview society' (Silverman 1997). This is due, in part, to the media saturation of interviews on television, radio and online, and it is 'as if interviewing is now part of the mass culture, so that it has actually become the most feasible mechanism for obtaining information about individuals, groups and organisations' (Fontana and Frey 2003: 64).

In relation to research, *qualitative interviewing* has become the most commonly used method for acquiring information about people's lives. This demonstrates the importance of interviewing in the field of youth research by indicating that, despite the emphasis on statistics in policy, individual experiences are perhaps becoming increasingly important.

Interviewing is a flexible method of obtaining data, allowing the researcher to study subjective viewpoints (Flick 2009). This interviewing process is underpinned by the belief that in-depth accounts of people's individual experiences and opinions are important. Ensuring that the voices of participants are heard and that the data are viewed through their eyes will allow the researcher to 'discover and do justice to their perceptions and the complexity of their interpretations' (Richards and Morse 2007: 30).

Research interviews utilised within the youth work setting are often conducted as part of evaluation research in order to assess programme delivery. Qualitative interviewing provides the opportunity to find out what project 'success' means to clients, staff and funders through exploration of the effectiveness of its output levels. It can also work to investigate those many aspects of project outcomes that pose methodological challenges to the researcher, such as whether a young person's aspirations have been raised. This outcome cannot be studied in isolation from the project, because it is likely to have been influenced by a number of other external factors.

## Different types of interview

In this section I shall provide a brief account of different forms of interview and different ways of asking questions. 'Interviewing . . . is not a research method but a family of research approaches that have only one thing in common – conversation between people in which one person has the role of researcher' (Askey and Knight 1999: 2).

## Structured interviews

This approach is more akin to a quantitative research method as the questions are similar to those found within a questionnaire. The researcher has tight control over the format of questions and answers, and each question is intended to be asked in the same way and order to minimise the influence of the investigator on the data collection process. Structured interviews contain predominantly closed rather than open questions that do not give scope for deviating from the topic. A closed question is one in which the answer is predetermined: for example, 'On a scale of 1 to 5, to what extent do you think having a youth work qualification improves a practitioner's practice?'

## Semi-structured interviews

The qualitative – semi-structured – interview is the most commonly used research method used with young people (Heath *et al.* 2009). A semi-structured interview is characterised by a defined topic and one of its advantages is that it allows respondents to answer on their own terms whilst the researcher can seek 'both clarification and elaboration' (May 2001: 123). The *semi-standardised* interview follows a set of main questions whose order can be changed by the researcher in order to probe for the most relevant information, as often questions from the schedule have already been answered during a response to previous questions. Interviewers may also ask participants to develop or expand answers for clarity. This prevents the interviews appearing stilted and formal. Ideally these interviews should be similar to a flowing conversation. This approach allows the interviewer to gather similar content matter from respondents with the purpose of defining similar themes, whilst also acknowledging the potential contradictions or differences between opinions and experiences. Open questions are utilised here: for example, 'In what ways does having a youth work qualification improve workers' practice?'

## Unstructured interviews

These interviews aim to explore fully interviewees' own understandings of a particular subject by posing general, open questions, such as: 'Please tell me about your experience of . . .' The respondent, rather than the researcher, drives the interview and guides the conversation by introducing topics that are meaningful to them. This is another useful approach for the beginning of a research project in order to elicit themes that may then drive the project in different ways. The collected data form a narrative or story rather than a set of questions and answers, as is the case in both the structured and semi-structured formats. If necessary, the researcher may intervene at appropriate moments to encourage the participant to continue, but, 'essentially, the person tells his/her story about an incident or situation and you, as the researcher, listen passively' (Kumar 2005: 124).

## Paired interviews

Interviewing respondents in pairs can create a less formal atmosphere than a one-to-one interview – particularly if you do not know the respondents. Generally, friends are paired in order to develop the type of data and stories that may be captured, through shared experiences and voicing agreement and disagreement about the chosen topic. This format can also acknowledge the importance of 'best friend' relationships, which may be especially useful amongst young women. As with the focus group format (see below), this allows for the discussion of particular events or experiences common to both young people. In Bradford and Hey's (2007: 599) study this approach was used 'in order for the young people to feel supported' and to gather 'pair talk data' to encourage the 'working out' of their views and experiences. In addition, this can be viewed as an ethical way to conduct research with young people, as power relations are less weighted towards the investigator.

## Focus groups

Focus groups offer a method of interviewing more than one person at a time and are useful for exploring service impact. Because of the large number of opinions generated, they are also useful in identifying broad ideas and emerging themes at the beginning of a research project. These can be used to inform an interview schedule (or a questionnaire) in order to highlight issues that are worth pursuing at a later point. Focus groups can be employed to collate group responses and gain insights into shared understandings. They are likely to elicit several perspectives in a short space of time, but may be difficult to set up in relation to finding a time and a place that are appropriate for all participants.

Focus groups encourage participants to question each other's views, which may create a more informal atmosphere than one-to-one interviewing. According to Flick (2009: 204), the moderator should 'create a liberal climate, facilitating members to contribute opening both their experiences and opinions'. The method aims to reveal similar and contradictory views and to generate richer responses by allowing participants to challenge one another's opinions. It is important to bear in mind that this format may also cause disagreements within the group that may need to be managed carefully by the facilitator. However, these disagreements might be indicative of important issues that the researcher may wish to pursue. Ideally, two researchers should be present during a focus group to manage and observe behaviour and anticipate pressure points, situations that are relatively commonplace in youth work practice. Certain participants who may have been discouraged from airing their views during an interview may feel more relaxed discussing the topic with their peers. Conversely, some young people may feel more reluctant to speak out in front of their peers. It is therefore important to offer all group members the opportunity to talk so that some participants' opinions are not drowned out or silenced by stronger individuals.

There is no ideal number of focus group participants as each situation varies according to individual personalities. Too few and the conversation may not be sufficiently rich in detail; too many and the content may not develop in sufficient depth. Another difficulty with overly large groups is that people tend to speak over one another, or the group can break into separate conversations. If group members know one another, existing dynamics will be present, and these should be taken into consideration by the facilitator. However, broadly speaking, about six people is a good number for a focus group. Heath *et al.* (2009) point out that, within youth research, focus group moderators will attempt to speak to groups who already know one another. The facilitator should try to break the ice for unfamiliar group members, and ensure that the respondents feel comfortable enough to express their opinions freely.

When carrying out focus groups, utilising stimulus material (such as images from magazines, objects or video clips) is a useful way to facilitate discussion (Barbour 2007). This is also a means of encouraging some interviewees who may be reluctant to contribute, as such provision can provide a clear focus for the group.

## Developing and designing questions

Whatever format of interviews you decide to undertake, your questions will be directly linked to your primary research question. Before reaching the interview stage of the research process, you will have:

- familiarised yourself with the literature on your chosen topic (Is there enough to form the basis of an assignment/report/project? If not, ensure you are confident enough in the way you theorise research to be able to draw on literature from another field to support your topic);
- developed your idea to form a primary research question from which to explore an area of interest;
- chosen the appropriate research method in order to investigate your topic: e.g. semi-structured or structured interviews;
- established secondary research questions in order to narrow down your topic and inform your interview schedule;
- identified any ethical issues that require attention, such as consent forms; and
- arranged interviews and begun the fieldwork.

## Creating the semi-structured interview schedule

The interview schedule is based on a clear list of questions to be answered but it should be flexible enough to allow other relevant themes to develop during the interview. Robson (1993: 237) compares the semi-structured interview schedule to a 'shopping list' that allows the researcher freedom to explore existing and surrounding issues and questions. It is very important to familiarise yourself with the relevant literature surrounding your topic. This will help ensure that your interview schedule is focused and based on the themes you intend to investigate in your research. Good knowledge of the literature helps you identify the key questions.

Rather than creating themes after data collection is complete, they should emerge before the fieldwork has begun. This knowledge usually stems from reviewing existing literature relating to your research questions. This is where theory should be used to provide the basis to the research, offering a guide to establishing questions. Interview questions are developed from the themes that have driven your primary and secondary research questions, in addition to the surrounding literature of your topic. The secondary questions listed below are derived from the primary research question of a project on 'cool' (and 'uncool') identities I conducted with Simon Bradford. They should not be confused with the interview schedule questions.

Primary research question:

- How do young people mobilise cool and uncool in their identity practices?

Secondary questions:

- What is cool?
- How influential is cool in their lives?
- Where is cool found? Is it at school, on the streets, within peer groups or online?
- What types of cool performance are utilised?
- What does coolness tell us about young people's identity?

It is important that interview questions developed from these secondary questions are easily comprehensible to your interviewees. Pay close attention to the type of language used and reduce any possible ambiguities that may arise as much as possible. Posing the questions to a friend or colleague may assist with this process, although a more common way to test questions is to conduct a small pilot study in advance of the final one in order to gauge interviewees' reactions. Such trial runs enable researchers to eliminate any questions that do not elicit rich, detailed responses from participants. Sometimes researchers will rewrite their questions or add prompts to the existing ones. Gillham (2009) notes that the order of questions may also be rearranged after conducting a pilot so that each one leads seamlessly on to the next in the form of a narrative. Silverman (2010: 336) describes this process as 'developing through trial and error'.

Do not try to cover too much or too little by asking too many or too few questions. Whilst it is useful to have a couple of back-up questions in the event of the interview being briefer than anticipated, use these only if you believe that you have not exhausted the subject because transcribing data is very time consuming. There should be a logical ordering of questions based on your main themes. Although an interview differs from a conversation, similar principles can apply in terms of a natural order of topics covered. Avoid asking unclear questions or using jargon and abbreviations that may alienate the interviewee if they are unfamiliar with such terminology. Be sensitive to leading and biased questions as these will impact on the data collected, even though such questions may tell you a lot about how the interviewee understands particular issues. Although you are likely to have preconceived ideas about your topic, it is important that your respondent does not feel under pressure to agree with your viewpoint.

## Asking questions

Asking questions and analysing responses are aspects of being a youth practitioner, although the sorts of questions asked by practitioners may be quite different from those asked in a research context, as may the reasons for asking them. In research, you may be interested in theoretical questions rather than, say, questions about the particular outcomes of a project or the circumstances of a young person or a group. Conversations and informal discussion, rather than formal interviews, are often the means of engaging with young people as youth practitioners. The research-based interviewer should have 'familiarity with modes of questioning, in order for the interviewer to devote his or her attention to the interview subject and the topic' (Kvale 2009: 134). This is gained from extensive reading on your chosen topic.

It is natural for both the interviewer and interviewee to be a little nervous or anxious, particularly if interviewing individuals whom you have not met before. The interviewee may be wondering what to expect and whether their views will be relevant. The interviewer may be concerned with the extent to which the data they are collecting will provide usable material in the research project. Being clear about what the respondent should expect, outlining the details of the project, and pointing out that they can stop the interview at any time should go some way to alleviating any apprehension on the interviewee's part. Creating an informal atmosphere can work to reduce the power dynamics which are inevitably present (between adults and young people, different genders or people from different racial backgrounds, for example) in the interview context.

Practically, there are ways in which you can elicit more information from your respondents:

- Introductory questions to establish rapport – initial straightforward questions help to overcome nervousness about the situation and set up the interview for future questions. Save the most important questions for later in the interview, after the respondent has 'warmed up'.
- Prompting the interviewee may encourage them to divulge more information, such as asking, 'Can you tell me more about that?', 'Why do you think that might be the case?' and, for clarification purposes, 'So, that I understand correctly, what you're saying is . . .'
- Allow enough time for responses as different people process information at different rates – a slow response may be a sign that they are thinking carefully about what you have asked them.
- Remaining silent might provide the respondent enough time to formulate a response and will also indicate that you would like them to expand on their point.
- Repeating the question and/or the last few words spoken by the interviewee will also encourage answers. Asking for an example to illustrate the point is a useful tool for obtaining rich data.
- Active listening (i.e. being really engaged with the respondent and the interview process) is very important so that the interviewee feels valued by the researcher – it involves responding to what is being said in the context of the interview and

reflecting upon it rather than solely relying on predetermined questions. This can also be achieved through nodding your head and acknowledging their responses by saying 'yes', 'OK', 'hmmm', and so on.

- 'Body language' is crucial to understanding communication. However, when you first start conducting interviews you may be too preoccupied with all the other elements of the process to notice it. Once you do, it will help you make sense of the views being expressed in the interview. Also reflect upon your own body language and how this may be read by participants.

## Sampling and access

Sampling is a crucial element of the successful research project because it is important that participants adequately reflect the research problem. Your research sample consists of the people you intend to approach for an interview, so decisions have to be made about who to include and exclude (clearly, you cannot interview everyone who might provide interesting data, so you have to make choices). Qualitative research samples do not claim to be completely representative although they tend to draw from a wide range of individuals. On the whole, it is important that members of the sample provide a 'good understanding of the issue under research' (Bryne 2004: 186). As a result, the importance here lies with respondents constructing individual stories and 'truthful' versions of their lives.

A *non-probability sampling approach* is associated with qualitative research, 'units are deliberately selected to reflect particular features of groups within the sample population' (Richie and Lewis 2003: 78). In addition, this approach encompasses a 'relevant range of people' but does not claim to cover the entire population (Mason 2002: 91). It is important to bear in mind that sampling is a flexible rather than a fixed process. Sometimes an initial sample size will be increased or decreased according to what is revealed during the fieldwork.

In the case of the structured interview the sample can be large: questions are predetermined and conducting the interview and analysing the data can take less time. The unstructured interview will elicit a lot of data about many different topics, so a smaller sample is commonly used. Semi-structured interviews are likely to be carried out with a sample number somewhere in between, as both the researcher and the participants drive them. Students often ask how many interviews they should conduct for their project. It is impossible to give a precise figure, as each project is different and the sample size depends on the type of data sought and the inevitable practical matters of time and resources. Sufficient numbers have been reached when 'those outside the sample might have a chance to connect to the experiences of those in it' (Seidman 1991: 45). Additionally, as a general rule, once you have reached 'saturation' point (i.e. when you find that material in the data is repeating itself), it is probably time to stop.

A *snowball sampling* approach that utilises existing contacts and networks is often used in qualitative interviewing. The interviewees then become informants, identifying further potential respondents. This might involve asking young people you are already in contact with to get involved in your study. They may then be able to suggest other people they know who could take part and increase the sample size. The qualitative underpinning of the sampling frame (the list of all possible members of a population from which the sample will be selected) allows for this degree of responsive flexibility. Bryne (2004) points to the importance of considering carefully how the sample is developing. Snowball sampling can build in 'security', according to Lee (1993, cited in Cohen *et al.* 2007), as the researcher trusts the contacts to deliver what they have agreed. It is then hoped that the introduced participants will also engage with the project on the same level.

A snowball sample might be appropriate when the researcher requires access to a population considered hard to reach, and it could be particularly useful when investigating illicit activity, such as drug taking or graffiti writing. This sampling approach is flexible and accommodates the introduction of new participants into the study where this is appropriate. When using a snowball method, it is important to acknowledge that members of the sample may have similar characteristics, such as a shared socio-economic background.

Also known as *judgement sampling*, the purposive 'sample structure is developed from the analysis and the material' of your project (Flick 2009: 142). It relies on the researcher deciding who will provide the most useful information for the study in terms of social categories and opinions on the subject matter. For example, if you are investigating gender difference and similarity, you can adopt a purposive sampling technique in order to achieve a proportionately mixed sample of young men and women. This is necessary to contact participants according to certain characteristics, such as gender.

One other sampling approach that you may find relevant to your work is *cluster sampling*, whereby you target groups of respondents in one setting, such as a classroom of students (Blaikie 2010). The main concern here is the rationale for excluding and including certain people or groups in relation to your research objectives.

*Convenience sampling*, as the name suggests, involves selecting participants who are most readily available to you: perhaps all situated in one location, such as a youth club or arts project. This approach is likely to be both time and cost effective, but it might result in 'poor quality data [that] lacks intellectual credibility' (Marshall 1996: 521). As you will be seeking out the experiences of particular groups of people, to avoid choosing participants completely at random, the researcher can elect to be guided by such characteristics as age and ethnicity.

More than one sampling frame can be adopted to represent the research question more appropriately. For instance, in terms of the 'cool' research mentioned earlier, both a snowball and a purposive approach were adopted. In this way respondents were accessed through existing contacts. Furthermore, as the study was concerned with gender relations, this method also set criteria in terms of interviewing similar numbers of young men and young women.

## Ethical considerations

Practitioners who are new to research will already be operating with a code of ethics. As Sercombe (2010: 58) points out, 'no code imaginable would be able to cover all the range of contexts, cultural groups and issues youth workers cover in a single day's work'. The research ethics guidelines are similar in that they provide a framework to which interviewers should adhere through the safeguarding of young people and workers. The British Sociological Association (BSA 2002) sets out the professional code of research conduct.

Clarification of the purpose of the interview and what is expected of informants is crucial to the interview process. It is also important to point out that there is an option for the interviewee to withdraw from the interview at any time. This is unlikely to happen unless someone is being interviewed about a very sensitive issue. 'Predicting discomfort or distress during the data-gathering process may be impossible' (Oliver 2010: 32), but one way to anticipate this is to conduct a pilot study. Robson (1993: 235) proposes that a 'cool-off' – a few undemanding questions at the end of the interview – can alleviate any tension that may have built up earlier.

A letter outlining the project's aims, stating where the research will be published and confirming that sources will be anonymised is a common method of gaining participants' informed consent. The confidentiality of interview discussions should also be highlighted when conducting research, although this cannot be assured after focus groups or paired interviews. To accommodate this, the researcher can control the discussion by attempting to reduce the disclosure of information that may be considered too sensitive for use in the research.

Power relations between interviewer and interviewee should always be a central consideration. If the interviews take place in youth clubs or respondents' homes, that should work towards creating a more informal atmosphere between interviewer and interviewee. However, Heath *et al.* (2009) point out that this is not always the case: a young person's home may not always be the most appropriate place for interviews as family or friends could interrupt the conversation verbally or alter responses simply by their presence. Such issues might also arise in the busy confines of a youth centre. It is important to bear in mind that ethics is an ongoing process through the research, and merely acquiring university or organisational clearance is insufficient in terms of considering this aspect of the project.

## Recording and transcribing the interview

An audio recording device is commonly used during interviews because this enables the researcher to transcribe the data verbatim. Jotting down notes to record body language and/or highlight key points in the interview that may be important for the analysis is also employed by some investigators. However, this has the potentially negative effect of making the interviewer appear less interested in what the respondent has to say. When engaging with young people every situation is different, so the researcher must adapt to it and choose the most appropriate way of recording their opinions. Always check your equipment – before and during – to ensure the interview is being recorded correctly. A good-quality, USB-based Dictaphone is the most effective way of recording; mobile phones should be used only in an emergency. It is usual for interview material to be transcribed into written text (either the entire interview or parts of it). 'When researchers speak of a transcript, they are referring to a mode of representing a piece of data that has been gathered' (Brown and Gibson 2009: 109). Note that as a rough guide, transcribing will take approximately four times the length of your recording, but of course this depends on such variables as the interviewer's typing speed and the clarity of the recording. You may opt for a full or partial transcription. If a group becomes chaotic, or they all start talking about what they had for dinner last night, then a time code in the left column and a simple coding in the transcript (for example: *inaudible – participants all talk over each other* or *Group discusses dinner 3.24–4.56)* can be a saviour. Recently, I transcribed a twenty-minute interview that produced 2,500 words – a considerable amount of data to amass in a relatively short period of time. This is one reason why your interview schedule should be as focused as possible, although you may still gather material that may not appear to be immediately relevant to your research problem.

## Interview skills

There are many skills involved in being an effective interviewer, as each brings 'different conversational styles to the task of interviewing unique participants on diverse topics, and approach[es] their work from a variety theoretical perspectives' (Roulston 2010: 115). Some of the basic requirements, many of which youth practitioners may already possess, are:

- knowing your subject matter;
- arranging interviews well in advance of the project deadline in case people drop out at the last minute;
- ensuring there is enough time for the transcribing, analysing and writing up (it generally takes longer than you think!);
- always being punctual – being made to wait may impact negatively upon the respondent's engagement with the interview;
- ensuring you let the respondent know the purpose and duration of the interview, and where the results will be published;
- active listening – picking up on what the interviewee has said and steering the conversation appropriately;
- tolerating silences and knowing when to be quiet yourself – some people will take longer than others to respond;
- being able to manage your emotions if interviewees are expressing opinions which are at odds with your own;
- being able to mediate conflict, as appropriate, within focus groups;
- considering whether an interviewee has provided you with an account of their experiences that may be designed to please you or to emphasise certain things and obscure others – be sceptical and remember that people tell their stories in all sorts of ways and for all sorts of reasons;
- responding through reflection about the most appropriate research methods to be used throughout the research process; and

• transcribing your own data to ensure familiarity throughout the research process. There are professional transcribers, but they may be unfamiliar with the specific language and vocabulary that young people, youth practitioners and others use to describe their experiences. In transcription notes consider including non-verbal material (e.g. facial expressions, giggles or noises), which may add richness to your analysis and will help you to interpret what has been said.

## Coding and analysis

Qualitative research may be primarily concerned with making generalisations or its purpose may be to explore in-depth individual stories. Stories or narratives provide the data that can then be analysed and will serve to drive the project and respond to the research questions. The forms of data that may be analysed in this way will include interviews, focus group sessions, field notes, personal diaries, observation logs, and so on. In fact, any kind of written material is amenable to the analysis outlined here.

Developing and analysing your data really begins with the literature review, which, in turn, informs how the interview schedule (your list of questions) is constructed and ordered. Having identified and studied the key texts, a number of common threads will start to become evident from the literature – we can refer to these as *themes*. It is the researcher's job to select which of these themes are most relevant to the research question. (However, you should remember that the literature may not have identified everything that is important in relation to a particular topic of study; there is always something that your work can add.) Selecting key themes can be based on what you want to know, your interests, number of previous studies, country of origin and so on in order to narrow the focus of the topic. You could concentrate on *predefined* themes that come from your reading or understanding of the literature, or you might want to look for *emergent* themes that you have spotted in the transcripts. Indeed, you might want to work with both of these, and you could combine them by starting with some predefined themes and then add some of the emergent themes.

There is no single or best way to analyse qualitative data, but you certainly need to be disciplined and systematic. During, and after, data collection you will begin to identify the emerging ideas (themes) from your data. These may mirror the themes that you have identified from the literature, but they will be more connected with your interests, as they will have emerged from *your* data rather than from existing theory. In other cases new, contradictory or dominant themes may become evident and you may choose to pursue these.

When you start to go through your transcriptions, remind yourself what you are interested in (go back to your research problem as that is the main guide to what it is that you want to learn). As you read through, you will identify ideas, words or phrases that emerge in the transcripts – we can refer to these as *codes*. Coding can be viewed as a preliminary part of the data analysis process. However, reading and rereading the data are necessary in order to identify these codes. The nature of coding is contested and therefore there is the 'potential for considerable confusion regarding what coding actually is' (Bernard and Ryan 2003: 218). During the initial coding process one is making 'assumptions about the kind of phenomena you are cataloguing and the kinds you are not' (Mason 2002: 148). Some data may fit more than one code or category. While coding is in some ways similar to completing a puzzle, in qualitative research there will always be overlapping data because material will often fit into more than one assigned code or will become part of more than one theme.

You can organise these codes into the groups that we call *themes*. I offer an example from the 'cool' identity project. In this case the data came from a series of semi-structured interviews with young people in which they were asked to talk about cool and being cool. These interviews were transcribed and the transcriptions read and reread to identify a number of codes that appeared across the mass of the data. The codes were then grouped to form a number of themes that, again, were evident throughouot the data. What you see below is a very preliminary attempt to put some order into the data so that we can begin to know something of how young people talk about and understand cool and uncool. The short extracts from the interviews are included so you can see the types of comments made by the young people. The codes in the left-hand column of Box 5.1 are the ideas, words and phrases that seemed important when I was reading through the transcripts of those interviews. You can underline or mark these on the extracts as you read through them (you could also give them numbers or abbreviations).

Byron: Being cool is not major. It's not a thing that you have to be, it's like you choose to be cool or not.

Shani: In school there's also pressure – the clothes you wear have to be labelled 'cos lots of people wear Nike and that's kind of cool because everyone is wearing it.

Alex: There's a bit of pressure if you're not current with your clothes or anything then you can fall back a bit and people have like a different perspective of you.

Tiya: I think it's a lot of pressure for other people but for me it's not.

Reena: With girls it's being girly. Maybe some girls who are considered cool would wear really short skirts with all the make-up on.

Naina: Yeah, some are quite smart and stuff but they'll give the image, make-up, fully done make-up.

Tiya: With the girly girls it's like 'Oh I need to do my hair properly, I need to do my make-up and everything.' I think that's kind of true with me as well. The boys it's just like jogging bottoms, some boys dress up, they spike their hair up and gel it every morning.

Naina: I think it's probably more with guys because guys will be like with their Ecco stuff . . . a lot of the whole new image is like trackies, low-cut jeans, hoodies, big baggy.

Katy: The boys and all that, if you're wearing Adidas and Nike and that yeah you're cool.

Jaden: For some people they take it seriously, they have to wear Nikes.

Ita: I know it's expensive and that but you feel good.

Once you have gone through your data in order to identify all the important codes and have refined the themes, they will provide the basis for your overall analysis. In completing that you should be looking at the relative significance of each overall theme (how

## Box 5.1  Codes and themes

| Codes | Themes |
|---|---|
| a) Cool is not so important; b) choosing cool; c) being pressured to be cool; d) clothes, fashion and cool; e) feeling good; f) subconscious cool | What counts as cool? |
| a) Girl cool is different from boy cool; b) really short skirts and make-up; c) for boys, being casual; d) trackies, hoodies, low-cut jeans | Gendered cool |
| a) Brands and cool; b) expensive; c) taking it seriously | Cool brands |

many times it appears in the data, for example); which main ideas or topics appear in each theme; possible linkages between themes that might give an overall pattern to the data. Note that neither the codes nor the themes are fixed, as you will continue refine them throughout the stages of your research project as you add more data and analyse the material further.

In order to do justice to your research data, it is vital to:

- understand the time-consuming nature of this stage of the research process – this stage of the analysis is very labour intensive;
- familiarise yourself with your transcribed data as this will speed up the analysis process – take it wherever you go and read, read, read;
- keep a copy of the transcriptions with you and go through the interviews systematically identifying codes, themes and sub-themes;
- accept that it is not possible to cover everything uncovered by the research so stick to the main themes during the analysis and writing-up stages;
- create headings of your themes in Word, and drag and drop the representative interview quotes into the appropriate sections; and
- save and back up all your work regularly – recoding the same data more than once is time-consuming.

The structure of the dissertation or report themes will determine the way in which your final piece of work is produced. It will probably be something like this:

- introduction;
- review of the literature;

- research design and methods;
- data analysis;
- interpretation; and
- conclusions.

The literature review and data analysis sections should be in a constant conversation with one another, as one supports the other. The purpose of the review is to introduce the texts which you will be analysing and contrasting in more depth later. Your analysis will then be split into chapters covering the main themes of your project. In addition to showcasing your data, you will be drawing on the literature that you introduced in the literature review section in a more in-depth way. Your findings will support and/or contradict what has already been said on your topic. It is your task to develop an argument in which you embed the interview responses within a theorised discussion based on the existing relevant literature.

## Opportunities, challenges and constraints of interviewing and analysing data

Interviewing offers much potential and opportunity for collecting rich and valuable data that can respond to a range of research questions. However, it does not (and cannot) do everything. In this section, the strengths and limitations of interviewing are identified, in particular the questions of reliability, validity and bias. These matters are often raised in relation to interviewing.

### *Reliability and validity*

As Golafshani (2003: 601) argues, to 'ensure reliability in qualitative research, examination of trustworthiness is crucial', because the reader has to rely on the researcher's interpretation of the interview data. The reliability of data relates to the consistency of the interview – would the results be similar if it were conducted by another interviewer using the same method? The idea of reliability comes from the natural sciences and is probably more appropriately applied to structured, rather than semi-structured (or unstructured), qualitative interviewing, as the former approach aims to minimise the impact of the investigator. Repeating a semi-structured interview will not necessarily elicit the same responses, content and phrasing will be different because 'social life is not repetitive or stable, and so our research perceptions of it cannot be entirely consistent' (Payne and Payne 2004: 198).

'Validity is another word for truth . . . How are they [researchers] to convince themselves (and their audience) that their "findings" are genuinely based on investigation,' asks Silverman (2010: 275–276). Validity, therefore, is concerned with the extent to which interview questions have been adequately developed in order to answer the research question at hand. Qualitative research relies on the interpretative qualities and skills of the researcher. As a result, the validity of this approach is reliant on careful consideration of the methodology being used and the degree to which the findings are an accurate interpretation of events. If qualitative interviews are social encounters (May 2001), researchers are inevitably guided by their own sense of self.

## Bias

Acknowledging the researcher's position and their relationship to the data is particularly important in qualitative research. Subjectivity (i.e. how one's biography and life experiences influence decisions made during the research) should be taken into consideration during both data collection and data analysis. Furthermore, the assumptions made by the researcher are mediated and made accountable through discussions around their subjectivity and reflexivity (i.e. a conversation with ourselves about how we are relating to the data according to our subjective viewpoint).

For example, the researcher should take into account how interviewees perceive them, how they viewed the participants, and what influence either of these might have had on the project. The way one constructs research questions and engages with the literature is something that the researcher must be mindful of even before the research begins.

Acknowledgement of reflexivity can work to limit the bias that is often associated with qualitative research. However, it is more than a question of reflecting; it is an 'element of self-study . . . and alerts researchers to the need to question the taken for granted knowledge they take into a study' (Richards 2009: 205). You will need to consider the relationship between subjectivity and reflexivity, and how this has impacted upon the entire research process. One effective way of doing this is to create a reflexive research diary that outlines important milestones or challenges experienced while collecting data. This is a very useful tool in engaging critically with the challenges of doing qualitative interviewing. For example, consider how the data make you *feel* and the impact this might have on the analysis. You may empathise more with a particular interviewee one day than another. It is important to acknowledge that mood may affect the analysis process. These are all examples of potential bias.

One way to limit such bias is to read and reread the data over a period of time so that the analysis is consistent. Our moods change daily and so might the way we read the data, so a few readings of the transcripts will help eliminate this and avoid situations such as favouring one interviewee's experiences over those of another. As producers of research often begin with a theoretical framework and a strong sense of the direction of the study, one must also be mindful of not seeing what one wants to see and omitting the data that might not seem to 'fit'.

## Practice-based task 5.1 Interviews

Record a variety of TV interviews, such as those that occur on news programmes, sports shows and chat shows. Watch the clips with these questions in mind:

- In what ways do interviewees behave differently in these interview settings?
- What are the differences in style between the interviewers?
- Which different approaches has the interviewer adopted?
- Is there a rapport between the two parties?
- Is there evidence of leading or biased questions?
- Who holds the power in these contexts, and to what effect?

# Evaluation research

The evaluation of services for young people is increasingly commonplace these days in the assessment of a project's perceived 'success' and, often, to secure the next round of funding. (You might include here various needs assessments, process evaluations or the kinds of summative evaluations that often conclude funded projects.) In financially stricken contexts, such as post-recession Britain, this is likely to become even more prevalent, as an inability to demonstrate value and outcome will inevitably mean no further funding. Funding bodies and policy-makers are extremely keen for providers to 'evidence' the effectiveness of practice-based interventions, often in relation to such indicators as reach of service (how many young people?), cost effectiveness or demonstrated effectiveness (perhaps measuring numbers of young people entering the job market or achieving accreditation). In order for a project to survive, therefore, effective evaluation becomes an essential part of practice.

The extent to which the anticipated (or required) outputs and outcomes of a project have been met is a common topic in evaluation research. Questions asked range from how well projects are achieving their aims to why they are succeeding and failing, whether they should be repeated with other groups, whether the project is cost effective, and how it might be improved with extra funding.

Practitioners are likely to have their own opinions about the extent to which a project is meeting its targets, what 'targets' means in the context of the programme delivery, and how young people are being treated by professionals and volunteers in the organisation as a whole. 'Proof' of the effectiveness of such programmes – and suggested ways of improving them – is derived through the process of evaluation research. Those involved may have very different ideas and perspectives about what counts as 'proof', and how it should be analysed and presented. Such evidence is likely to differ widely. For one youth worker, it might be a young person completing accreditation; for another, it could be watching them become more socially competent or confident. Evaluation research works to 'inform decision makers about the state of play of a current or intended programme of actions . . . The purposes vary from the attempts to improve performance and accountability through to social critique and transformation' (Schostak 2006: 24).

The Social Return on Investment (SROI 2004: 3.1) suggests that evaluation is concerned with the way social outputs are measured – that is, how the value of a particular intervention's social objectives might be calculated. It identifies two of the key elements in the evaluation process as *outputs* and *outcomes*. The former are 'a direct result of your programme goal . . . for example 25 people learned new computer skills', while the latter comprise a 'change that has occurred over the long term. So, for example, the number of people who started work and improved their personal circumstance.' Either or both of these may be important, depending on the intentions of the evaluation itself. Again, clear criteria and purposes are necessary from the beginning.

The evaluation tends to be measured against existing stated project outcomes. However, these outcomes may be interpreted in different ways by funders, stakeholders, managers, workers and young people. Are these outcomes short term, long term, local or national? Green and South (2006: 62) note the 'importance of clear objectives in defining success and establishing appropriate indicators'. The collaboration of projects with similar but distinct agendas, such as combating racism and crime reduction initiatives, can also render the identification of a core agenda problematic. Evaluation research differs from other types of research in that the researcher does not set the research agenda; rather, this tends to be done by funders or managers. Recommendations can be made for further research to be conducted in those areas that are of interest but not previously identified.

## How are ambiguous outcomes measured?

There is often an emphasis in quantitative research to demonstrate whether outcomes have been met. However, qualitative research often works to explore new areas of interest or the so-called 'softer' indicators of effectiveness. Quantitative methods are most commonly used and expected by funders and/or policy-makers, as they have traditionally been understood as having more credibility than qualitative research. So-called 'hard' data are often valued because they appear to give a clearer and less ambiguous answer to questions to which funders demand responses. Qualitative research can be used to explore 'fuzzy' evaluation outcomes whose effectiveness is not straightforward (Green and South 2006: 129). The qualitative interview perspective becomes key, then, in exploring programme objectives that 'focus upon involvement and personal achievement rather than dubious claims relating to causality' (Crabbe 2005: 7).

Measuring the 'success' of a project is complicated, given that politicians, managers, workers and young people define it in potentially very different ways. This type of evaluation demands that researchers understand the politics, complexity and ambiguity of evaluation. Project success is linked to the personal goals of the individual clients or users and the success of the project as a whole. One young person taking part in a regular activity may be considered to indicate success by one partner, while another might recognise success in the way the young people in a project are engaging with peers and developing social skills. Ideas of success, then, can be 'socially shared', and the way in which practitioners try to work towards some agreements is crucial in the process of evaluation. If outcomes are measured simply by numbers of young people attending sessions, that metric does not account for those who have benefited from the project but no longer turn up. Furthermore, attendance does not necessarily equate to positive engagement, as some young people might turn up but refuse to participate. If success were to be measured by numbers attending (and that *might* be a legitimate indicator), a measure of time would need to be identified and agreed in terms that constitute 'success'.

Evaluating a smoking cessation project may thus be far more straightforward than a programme that aims to broaden the horizons of local young people. The number of people who have given up smoking (or at least say they have) can be compared to the overall group to illustrate the effectiveness of such a programme. But measuring success in youth work programmes is much more complex as it is concerned with much more ambiguous issues: emotions, understandings and perceptions, for example – the so-called 'softer' indicators. However, it is entirely possible to make judgements about these, providing care is taken in defining the criteria for those judgements.

## Differences between internal and external evaluations

Internal or external evaluators can conduct evaluations. One motivation for internal evaluation is the level of staff knowledge about the organisation and its clients that can be exploited in the evaluation itself. Another motivation for internal research and evaluation is often financial: it can be expensive to fund a research project undertaken by external evaluators. On the other hand, it can be very difficult for internal staff to be independent and not take elements of what they observe or hear for granted. Existing allegiances and relationships may also influence how the data are collected and analysed. There may well be expectations from colleagues that one of their peers would not report on their practice in a negative way. It would be more risky still for a worker to report that senior staff are not doing their job properly, or to criticise other senior members of the team. Another consideration is the objectivity of insider research. Questions may be asked about the impartiality of the interviewer if the outcome of their enquiries determines whether their organisation receives further funding. So, there are serious questions here about credibility and the authority of research and evaluation.

External evaluation projects will take time and money to establish, and may include waiting time to secure a bid to acquire funding. However, the investigators will be trained in conducting research and will bring 'fresh eyes' to the situation, and this is sometimes considered to be a more credible approach. External evaluators are often thought to be more *objective* about what they see. Reporting negative feedback will always need to be approached carefully (in both insider and external research and evaluations), but feedback (or indeed feed-forward) is a crucial part of the evaluation process. It is important at the start of any evaluation that roles are defined and agreed by the stakeholders and then passed to each member of staff so that everyone is clear about these matters from the outset.

One of the possible negative aspects of external evaluation is that the interests of the project and its staff may not necessarily receive priority over those of stakeholders and funders. External evaluators 'may also be seen as intimidating by project staff, whatever their personalities and ways of working' (Green and South 2006: 9). One way to limit the effects of such suspicion is to carry out research *with* rather than *on* practitioners and clients. By adopting a participatory action research (PAR) approach (see Chapter 1), the aim is to bring about positive change through collaboration. Judgements will have to be made about how realistic this might be in any particular organisation and, once again, the politics of evaluation are likely to be present.

## Practice-based task 5.2  Evaluations

- Consider how your previous or current youth practice context evaluates and develops practice.
- Do you use insider or outsider evaluators?
- What parts of the programme and projects are evaluated?
- What methods are used? Why use these methods rather than others? Are they the most appropriate to answer the scope of the evaluation?

## Case study 5.1

## Sport interventions and young people

I was part of a Positive Futures (PF) evaluation project funded by the Home Office. A team of researchers worked in collaboration for two years on the largest piece of social policy research ever conducted on youth work and sport interventions. Extensive ethnographic fieldwork was carried out at national PF projects, which aimed to broaden the horizons of ten–nineteen-year-olds from areas identified by the government as 'deprived'. Being a complex outcome, consequently, much of this involved qualitative methods, such as observations and interviewing, all of which was underpinned by a participatory framework. In this way young people and workers in the field were regarded as stakeholders in the research.

Green and South (2006: 6) acknowledge that recently 'evaluation has become more integrated within programme delivery and is more likely to involve practitioners themselves'. What has helped the programme 'to set the pace amongst youth oriented social inclusion programmes is its consistent and on-going commitment to being informed by a robust research and evidence base' (Crabbe 2008).

Part of the research and evaluation remit was to identify how youth workers build positive relationships with young people through physical activities and sport. Investigating such concepts as 'cool', 'respect' and 'cultural intermediaries' (Crabbe 2005) necessitated the choice of a qualitative approach. I attended sessions and took on the role of youth worker in order to explore how these relationships were developed. Prior to starting the fieldwork, I decided that semi-structured interviews would be the ideal method to obtain the type of data I was looking for. Whilst this was the case when speaking to certain young people, others found the questions and recording equipment used in interviews too formal and became self-conscious. As a response to this, more informal chats whilst hanging out at sessions became the most useful source of data. Interviews worked well with most of the staff, allowing me to cover a lot of ground in a relatively short time.

Thus, a flexible approach to research is important, as a research field can never be wholly anticipated, and it is often best finalised once fieldwork has begun. Whilst some organisations may be resistant to this approach, many understand that research is a process that is context specific and carried out in a different way each time it is undertaken.

## Summary of key points

- There are different types of qualitative interview: the most commonly used with young people is the semi-structured method.
- There is a variety of sampling techniques (*convenience, snowball, judgement*). Take some time considering your technique, as the sampling frame and size of sample you choose will have significant impact on your research project.
- Piloting interview questions and approach can support interviewers in developing an effective interview approach. Bear in mind the need to consider the number of participants, the location and duration of interviews, and method of recording before commencing with the research.
- A qualitative interviewer should explain the kinds of account and the claims for the data, and personal bias when interpreting data.
- Evaluations are a key part of reflecting upon and developing policy and practice. Whilst quantitative approaches are often used in evaluations of practice contexts, qualitative methods can complement and develop evaluation processes in many contexts.
- Measuring ambiguous entities, such as 'success', or demonstrating clear changes in conduct or understanding may be challenging in many youth practice contexts. Blended, mixed method approaches using both qualitative and quantitative techniques can enable evaluators to provide indicators and richer qualitative data to support and evidence work within youth practice contexts.

## Practice-based task 5.3  Evaluating a project

You have been asked to conduct some evaluation research by the head of service to identify the extent to which young people's aspirations have been raised by a locally funded sports, arts or music youth project. First, you need to identify the project outcomes and decide which you intend to focus on for the purpose of your evaluation. The mapping of these outcomes will inform your chosen methodological framework.

Choose *one* (sports, arts or music) of the three projects and ask yourself:

- What are the challenges of this type of research?
- How would you begin to measure 'raised aspirations'?
- Which research methods would you use and why?
- Which people, and how many, would you speak to?
- Are there ethical issues to address?
- How will you analyse the data?
- How might your findings shape future projects?

## Further reading

There are many useful texts that can support you in designing and analysing interview approaches. Here are some I would recommend:

Green, J. and South, J. (2006) *Evaluation*, Maidenhead: Open University Press.
Kvale, S. (2009) *Doing Interviews*, London: Sage.
Mason, J. (2002) *Qualitative Interviewing*, London: Sage.
Richards, L. (2009) *Handling Qualitative Data*, London: Sage.

## References

Allen, G. and Langford, D. (2008) *Effective Interviewing in Social Work and Social Care*, Basingstoke: Palgrave.
Askey, H. and Knight, P. (1999) *Interviewing for Social Scientists*, London: Sage.
Barbour, R. (2007) *Doing Focus Groups*, London: Sage.
Bergman, M. (2008) *Advances in Mixed Methods Research*, London: Sage.
Bernard, R. and Ryan, G. (2003) 'Techniques to Identity Themes', *Field Methods*, 15(1): 85–109.
Blaikie, N. (2010) *Designing Social Research*, Cambridge: Polity Press.
Bradford, S. and Hey, V. (2007) 'Successful Subjectivities? The Successification of Class, Ethnic and Gender Positions', *Journal of Education Policy*, 22 (6): 595–614.
Brown, A. and Gibson, W. (2009) *Working with Qualitative Data*, London: Sage.
Bryne, B. (2004) 'Qualitative Interviewing', in C. Searle (ed.), *Researching Culture and Society*, London: Sage.

BSA (2002) *Statement of Ethical Practice for the British Sociological Association.* http://www.britsoc.co.uk/equality/Statement+Ethical+Practice.htm (accessed 24 November 2010).

Cohen, L., Manion, L. and Morrison, K. (2007) *Research Methods in Education*, London: Routledge.

Crabbe, T. (2005) *Getting to Know You: Engagement and Relationship Building*, London: Home Office.

Crabbe, T. (2008) *Youth Anti-crime Programme Sees Increase in Participation.* http://www.supportsolutions.co.uk/forum/viewtopic.php?f=24andt=2636andstart=0 (accessed 21 November 2010).

Flick, U. (2009) *An Introduction to Qualitative Research*, London: Sage.

Fontana, A. and Frey, J. (2003) 'The Interview: From Neutral Stance to Political Involvement', in N. Denzin and Y. Lincoln (eds), *Collecting and Interpreting Qualitative Materials*, London: Sage.

Gibb, G. (2007) *Analysing Qualitative Data*, London: Sage.

Gillham, B. (2009) *Research Interviewing*, Maidenhead: Open University Press.

Golafshani, N. (2003) 'Understanding Reliability and Validity in Qualitative Research', *Qualitative Report*, 8 (4): 597–607.

Green, J. and South, J. (2006) *Evaluation*, Maidenhead: Open University Press.

Grinnell, F. (2001) *Social Work and Evaluation Research: Quantitative and Qualitative Approaches*, Monument, CO: Peacock.

Heath, S., Brooks, R., Cleaver, E. and Ireland, E. (2009) *Researching Young People's Lives*, London: Sage.

Kumar, R. (2005) *Research Methodology*, London: Sage.

Kvale, S. (2009) *Doing Interviews*, London, Sage.

Marshall, M. (1996) 'Sampling for Qualitative Research', *Family Practice*, 13: 522–525.

Mason, J. (2002) *Qualitative Interviewing*, London: Sage.

May, T. (2001) *Social Research: Issues, Methods and Process*, Maidenhead: Open University Press.

Oliver, P. (2010) *The Student's Guide to Research Ethics*, Maidenhead: Open University Press.

Payne, G. and Payne, J. (2004) *Key Concepts in Social Research*, London: Sage.

Richards, L. (2009) *Handling Qualitative Data*, London: Sage.

Richards, L. and Morse, M. (2007) *User's Guide to Qualitative Methods*, London: Sage.

Richie, J. and Lewis, J. (2003) *Qualitative Research Practice*, London: Sage.

Robson, C. (1993) *Real World Research*, Oxford: Blackwell.

Roulston, K. (2010) *Reflective Interviewing: A Guide to Theory and Practice*, London: Sage.

Schostak, J. (2006) *Interviewing and Representation in Qualitative Research*, London: Sage.

Seidman, I.E. (1991) *Interviewing as Qualitative Research: A Guide for Researchers in Education and the Social Sciences*, New York: Teachers College Press.

Sercombe, H. (2010) *Youth Work Ethics*, London: Sage.

Silverman, D. (1997) 'Kundera's *Immortality*: The Interview Society and the Invention of the Self', *Qualitative Inquiry*, 3 (3), 304–325.

Silverman, D. (2010) *Doing Qualitative Research*, London: Sage.

SROI (2004) *Measuring Social Impact: The Foundation of Social Return on Investment.* http://www.neweconomics.org (accessed 9 October 2010).

# 6 Using quantitative methods

## Designing surveys and evaluations

Marilyn Clark and Albert Bell

## Overview

Youth research is dynamic and trans-disciplinary. It comprises myriad areas of interest, practices and methods. Youth practitioners are increasingly required to engage in survey or evaluation research to demonstrate the value of their work. Evidence-based practice has become a powerful movement and is now a core element of many governments' approaches to policy-making and youth work intervention. However, its emergence has generated much debate and raised challenging questions, particularly in relation to the interface between research, policy and practice (Chisholm 2006). This chapter will provide youth workers with the tools to engage effectively with quantitative research methods as part of their practice. Chisholm (2006: 23) maintains that '[r]esearchers and practitioners inhabit different cultural spaces' and it is a challenge to develop ways for both parties to cross these cultural spaces.

Practitioner-researchers perform a dual role. Since their research involvement is often small-scale, it is sometimes not defined as research. However, as Hargreaves (1996: 105) has aptly pointed out 'ways need to be found of legitimising [practitioner research], codifying it, and making it public'. Brooker and Macpherson (1998) contend that such research becomes useful when the research is informed by sound, 'scientific' practices. Changes in the world of work – with an increased emphasis on reflective practice – encourage practitioner research (Jarvis 1999). However, practitioner research may not be seen as *proper* research within academic or policy-making circles. It will only be taken seriously if practitioner researchers can be seen to have the requisite skills to conduct robust research that satisfies the rigorous requirements of the social scientific community. One may also argue that practitioners have more knowledge of practice than external researchers, so their research may be more insightful. 'The research community defines the epistemologies of research and also controls its image . . . But it is clear that both the traditional image and the new conception of research are already undergoing change' (Jarvis 1999: 7).

In the social sciences, including the youth field, there has been much complex discussion and argument around the topic of research methodology and how enquiry should proceed. There has probably been more energy expended on the debate on the relative advantages of qualitative and quantitative methods than almost any other methodological topic. Much of this debate centres on the issue of qualitative versus quantitative enquiry – which might be the better and which is more 'scientific'. Different methodologies become popular at different social, political, historical and cultural times and all methodologies have their strengths and weaknesses. Quantitative and qualitative research both rest on rich and varied traditions that come from multiple disciplines. While this chapter deals with the use of quantitative methods, youth practitioners are warned not to fall into the trap of thinking that quantitative research is 'better ' than qualitative research. While quantitative methods feature highly in service evaluation and needs assessment, and are highly valued in the current audit culture that surrounds youth work, it is not the case that quantitative research alone equals 'proper' research. The heart of the quantitative–qualitative debate is philosophical, not methodological.

While this text is about demonstrating the worth of quantitative and qualitative research as valid aspects of rigorous enquiry, this chapter will provide youth practitioners with the knowledge and skills to carry out quantitative research effectively. Quantitative research generates numerical data or data that can be converted into numbers and easily quantified. For quantitative researchers, a 'scientific' approach implies investigating a research problem deductively, whereby a hypothesis is formulated in terms of variables and tested by collected numerical data on each variable and analysed with statistical procedures. This operationalisation and measurement of variables allows for objective analysis.

This chapter will identify the main approaches to survey data collection. In particular, it will explore the advantages and limitations of surveys. The chapter will consider the relative strengths of cross-sectional and longitudinal survey designs, paying attention to issues of sampling, questionnaire design, reliability and validity. Research ethics will also be briefly considered in relation to quantitative research methodology and social surveys.

## Survey research methodology: origins and key concepts

Before undertaking a research project, whether this is engaged in as part of practice or as part of a commissioned study, the youth practitioner is faced with the inevitable choice of a research design. This choice involves certain philosophical assumptions about what constitutes knowledge, and implies a set of procedures or strategies of enquiry. It also includes detailed practices of data collection, analysis and report writing (Creswell 2003). Crotty (1998, cited in Creswell 2003) suggests that researchers should ask themselves four important questions at the planning stage of a research project:

1   *What theory of knowledge informs the research?* In the case of survey studies, objectivism – the notion that an objective reality exists and can be researched – is normally the underlying epistemology.

2  *What is the philosophical background behind the methodology in question?* In the case of surveys and other quantitative methods this is normally post-positivism (a reliance on the scientific method, with some reservations) characterised by social determinism (that is, the belief that human behaviour is the product of external social forces), reductionism (reducing the understanding of complex relationships to simple cause-and-effect relationships), empirical observation and measurement.

3  *What choice of methods will consequently be made?* The choice of methods for a quantitative researcher includes census studies, experiments and social surveys. This chapter is concerned with the use of surveys, which leads us to the next question.

4  *What research instruments, techniques and procedures are used?* Through questionnaire surveys, researchers look for data on predetermined variables and engage in statistical analysis.

According to Robinson (1998: 2), the basic ideals of logical positivism inform the quantitative approach in the social sciences, implying that knowledge is neutral and that standards of accuracy and precision offer a standardised, uniform framework for the generation of scientific knowledge. In its classic mould, positivism advanced the notion that the legitimacy of sociological enquiry depends on how effectively it embraces and applies the rigour of the natural sciences (Swingewood 2000).

Early positivists like the French sociologists Auguste Comte and Emile Durkheim contended that explanations of human conduct should be objective and scientific, and thus derived through systematic observation, comparison, measurement and quantification. These remain central to the quantitative approach, like social survey research. In contrast, the philosophical outlook that most informs *qualitative* research upholds the idea that sociological enquiry, by its very nature, can only be interpretative and cannot aspire towards the generation of generalisable explanations of human and social behaviour. Qualitative researchers thus tend to look quite sceptically at attempts to explain social behaviour through rigid and restrictive quantitative studies.

The positivistic philosophy of quantitative methods has also been criticised even within youth studies. Wyn and White (2008), for example, state that it does not examine issues in their wider socio-political and process contexts and that it is utilitarian and functional. However, we argue that such research, in combination with more qualitative and process accounts of young people's lives, is able to produce holistic knowledge and to consider 'commonalties' of experience. Quantitative research methodologies are often dictated by the strict canons of science, those of objectivity, controllability and replicability (i.e. repeatable by another researcher) and can help the youth practitioner move beyond popular conceptions of young people. People make confident claims about youth, such as that they use more mind-altering substances than were used in the past, or that youth crime is on the increase. However, as Coolican (1990) maintains, these notions may be 'hunches' masquerading as facts. The ever-growing demand for evidence-based approaches is the dominant rhetoric in policy-making circles. This may be a consequence of audit-driven government agencies and departments. It is, however, a reality that politicians and policy-makers want hard numbers to 'prove' the issues they wish to push forward. Because of this, quantitative research continues to be very widespread within policy and practice arenas. Statistical data are seen as 'factual', 'scientific', 'impartial' and evidencing an unassailable truth. However, statistical data are constructed in the same way as other forms of knowledge and can never be value free.

While it is important to take stock of all this, practitioner-researchers in the youth sector must also be aware of the strengths of quantitative research studies, including, most notably, survey research.

## Survey methods: advantages and limitations

The 'survey approach' refers to methods that emphasise quantitative analysis. Surveys normally take the form of close-ended questionnaires (such as the ESPAD survey questionnaire; see Case study 6.1 at the end of this chapter) and are usually paper-and-pencil instruments where the respondent anonymously completes a set of predetermined questions. Open-ended questions may also be included. According to Punch (2005), the word 'survey' has different meanings. Descriptive surveys describe samples in simple percentages and proportions and are often used in market or political research. They provide a 'snapshot' of the situation at a certain point in time. In social research, however, correlational surveys are more common. Correlations explain the level of association between two or more variables, such as the association between exposure to TV violence and increased youth crime, or the relationship between the age of first use of a substance and patterns of use. A variable is anything that varies. To say that two variables are related is to say that they vary together or share a 'common variance'. Coolican (1990) writes that the scope of scientific research is to relate changes in some variables to changes in other variables. So, for example, gender is an important variable to measure in terms of involvement in crime. Males are overrepresented in crime statistics, so any examination of criminality needs to take gender into consideration.

Some examples of surveys in youth and community studies may be found in Box 6.1.

---

### Box 6.1  Examples of UK surveys

- *A national survey of problem behaviour and associated risk and protective factors among young people*. This survey of 14,000 UK school students (Years 7–11) assessed involvement in crime, drug and alcohol misuse and other forms of problematic behaviour as well as factors associated with greater exposure to risk (Beniart *et al.*, 2002). See http://www.jrf.org.uk/publications/national-survey-problem-behaviour-and-associated-risk-and-protective-factors-among-youn.
- *Youth Lifestyles Survey, 1998*. This household survey measured self-reported offending of twelve–thirty-year-olds in England and Wales. It was first conducted in 1992 among fourteen–twenty-five-year-olds by Graham and

---

Bowling (entitled 'Young People and Crime Survey') and was repeated in 1998 to establish changes in trends and patterns of youth offending and desistance factors with the aim of establishing whether self-reported youth offending had changed since the first sweep in 1992 (see Graham and Bowling, 1995). See http://rds.homeoffice.gov.uk/rds/pdfs/r127.pdf.

- *Youth Cohort Study: Activities and Experiences of 17-Year-Olds: England and Wales, 2005.* This study includes a series of longitudinal surveys involving a sample of a young people following completion of statutory schooling and usually annually until they are aged nineteen or twenty. It examines participants' transition from school to work, how their skills match labour market demands and other issues. See http://www.education.gov.uk/rsgateway/DB/SFR/s000619/index.shtml.

## Practice-based task 6.1  Youth crime

Review the results from the Cambridge Study in Delinquent Development and identify the main risk variables for involvement in youth crime. See http://www.library.carleton.ca/ssdata/surveys/doc/pdf_files/csdd-uk-61-81-cbk.pdf. What are the problems associated with a risk paradigm approach in youth research?

## Generalisability and other crucial matters

By generalisability, most quantitative researchers understand that one is able to say that one's findings can be applied 'beyond the confines of the particular context in which the research was conducted' (Bryman 2008: 156). So, for example, if a youth worker were to conduct a study on the leisure patterns of a representative sample of young people in a particular context, we might want to consider how the observations drawn from this study might be 'generalised' beyond that particular sample group.

The concern with generalisability emerges in survey research, and attention is given to the question of how one can have a *representative* sample. The use of large representative samples allows for greater confidence in the generalisability of the results (Jick 1983: 138). In attempting to understand youth trends, surveys are useful in describing the characteristics of large populations, a capability not shared by other methods. For example, in the ESPAD survey, very large samples are used. Large samples minimise 'sampling error'. In statistics, sampling (or estimation) error is the error caused by observing a sample instead of the whole population. Vidich and Shapiro (1955: 31, cited in Gable 1994) highlight the superior 'deductibility' of the survey method over field methods that normally value validity over representation and generalisability.

According to Attewell and Rule (1991: 313, cited in Gable 1994) 'traditional survey work is strong in . . . areas where field methods are weak'. However, Bryman (2008: 157) warns against the temptation to over-generalise, or 'to see findings as having a more pervasive applicability . . . The concern to be able to generalize is often so deeply ingrained that the limits to the generalisability of findings are frequently forgotten or side stepped.'

Surveys allow many questions to be asked about a given topic, giving considerable scope and flexibility to the analysis. For example, the ESPAD survey measures leisure, patterns of substance use, peer group affiliations and many other variables, potentially allowing a multitude of relationships to be established. Survey studies have high reliability because standardised questions make measurement more precise by enforcing uniform definitions upon the participants. However, this may also be conceptualised as one of the weaknesses of this form of research in that it imposes a set worldview on the participants and does not allow them to explore their reality in their own terms, which contributes to diminished validity.

So, for example, when a survey questionnaire lists five possible reasons why young people use drugs and asks them to tick one of the options, it may omit alternatives not considered in the list. Kaplan and Duchon (1988: 572) suggest that '[t]he stripping of context [e.g. reduced "representability" or model complexity through the use of a closed survey instrument] buys "objectivity" and testability at the cost of a deeper understanding of what actually is occurring'. Surveys may be an uneasy fit with particular topic areas, such as in relation to studies trying to examine and understand meaning-making and the multifaceted nature of personal experience. In these examples, a qualitative research design may be much more appropriate. Moreover, while questions in surveys are general enough to be minimally appropriate for all respondents, this might miss what is most appropriate to many respondents, thereby reducing the validity of the survey itself.

The rigidity of using a set instrument throughout the data collection process gives survey research relatively poorer 'discoverability' when compared to more flexible and inductive methods. Once the work is under way, there is little one can do upon realising that some crucial item was omitted from the questionnaire, or upon discovering that a question is ambiguous or misunderstood by respondents. This makes piloting the research instrument prior to starting data collection critical for the success of one's study. Once a research instrument (your questionnaire) is adequately piloted, it is essential that it retain uniformity when administered, as reliability and generalisability would be otherwise impaired. You may want to pilot a short survey about young people's spending habits with a small group before rolling it out to all young people attending schools and youth centres in a town. Keeping the same questions and scales throughout the data collection process ensures standardisation. Standardised, tried and tested research instruments allow for comparisons through time. The same instrument may be used on another occasion in order to see if trends in youth lifestyles have changed. This emphasis on uniformity and standardisation in survey research contrasts with more qualitative approaches, particularly grounded theory, where the research instrument is changed to ensure that the participants' views are effectively captured.

# Reliability and validity

Reliability refers to the consistency of a measure of a concept and hence is an important consideration for any researcher intending to utilise a survey design (Black and Champion 1976; Bryman 2008; Johnston and Pennypacker 1980).

Reliability is ensured by consistency in procedures and evidenced by consistency in the reactions of research participants. If a research finding can be repeated, it is reliable. Repeating a research study to check for reliability is called replication using a standardised procedure. Validity implies truth: that is, whether the research instrument (the questionnaire, for example) measures what it is intended to measure. As Schutt (1999: 18) contends, researchers reach 'the goal of validity' when their 'statements or conclusions about empirical reality are correct'. Let us look at these two crucial constructs in more detail.

The above definitions clearly show that the construct of reliability is intimately tied to a study's degree of replicability: that is, the extent to which a measure, procedure or instrument yields the same result on repeated occasions. According to Bryman (2008), three main issues must be taken into account when considering whether a measure is reliable: stability, internal reliability and inter-observer consistency (not relevant to survey research but a major issue in content analysis). For a measure to be stable across different temporal contexts, the results relating to that measure for a particular group of respondents should not fluctuate over time. *Test–retest* reliability entails replicating the study under the same conditions and checking for differences in results. Testing for the reliability of a research tool using a similar but alternative tool (for example including questions on the same topics but ordered differently) is referred to as *alternative forms* reliability. The key issue with internal reliability is the extent to which the scores on one indicator are related to the scores of another, but related, indicator in the same scale. *Internal consistency* reliability controls for reliability in a questionnaire by grouping questions on the same topic into different sets and running correlation tests on the responses to these sets of questions.

A much-cited definition of validity is that of Hammersley (1987: 75): 'An account is valid or true if it represents accurately those features of the phenomena that it is intended to describe, explain or theorise.' So, for example, does a self-esteem measure really measure how an individual rates herself? A method can be reliable, consistently measuring the same thing, yet not valid. Validity thus comprises both *external validity* and *internal or causal validity*. External validity refers to the extent to which the results of a study are generalisable or transferable and is concerned with the degree to which research findings can be applied to the 'real world' beyond the controlled setting of the research. *Internal validity* refers to the rigour with which the study was conducted (for example, the study's design, the care taken to conduct measurements, and decisions concerning what was and was not measured) and the extent to which the designers of the study have taken into account alternative explanations for any causal relationships they explore (Huitt 1998; Schutt 1999). Attempts to increase internal validity are likely to reduce external validity as the study is conducted in a manner that is increasingly unlike the real world. Validity implies reliability: a valid measure must be reliable. But reliability does not necessarily imply validity: a reliable measure need not be valid (Bryman 2008).

Many critics have argued that quantitative research and the positivistic epistemology that guides it generally fail to make a distinction between the physical and the social world and the fact that people interpret and experience the world around them subjectively. In this respect, quantitative research, with its emphasis on direct observation, value neutrality, replication, uniformity, reliability and standardisation, is less attuned than qualitative research to study individual subjectivities. This task may prove difficult for quantitative researchers who would find immersion in subjective life-worlds not only a difficult prospect but possibly undesirable and 'unscientific'. This once again boils down to the argument that people place meaning on the world around them (Cicourel 1964: 108). Bryman (2008) also proposes that the dependence on instruments and procedures aimed at increasing reliability may actually hinder the connection between research and everyday life. The focus on the analysis of relationships between 'variables' also presents a static view of social life that is not reflective of reality.

Throughout the foregoing section we have identified the strengths and weaknesses of survey research. Table 6.1 summarises the main points mentioned above.

## Practice-based task 6.2  Reliability and validity

A youth worker colleague has devised a research tool to measure 'Attitudes of young people towards alcohol', which s/he wishes to administer to a group of young people in your youth club:

- How could the test be validated?
- How could the test be checked for reliability?

## Cross-sectional versus longitudinal designs

By the very nature of their field of study, youth researchers are concerned with change that occurs over time. This fact brings to light another research design choice that must be considered: longitudinal research versus cross-sectional research. Longitudinal research involves collecting data on the same people over time, while cross-sectional studies involve collecting data on different people at the same, fixed point in time. As longitudinal studies involve studying the same group of participants across a period of time, researchers are able to test hypotheses relating to cause and effect. It is contented that longitudinal studies are substantially free from reinterpretation of remembered information. They also provide the means to assess direction of effect (Tonry *et al.* 1991). The Cambridge Study in Delinquent Development (1961–1981) is a classic example of this sort of research. This study, initiated by Donald J. West and continued

**Table 6.1 Survey research: strengths and limitations**

| Strengths | Limitations |
| --- | --- |
| Normally quite inexpensive. | The generality of questions means that they may not be appropriate for all respondents. |
| Can describe the characteristics of a large population. Large samples are possible because of low cost, increasing the likelihood that the results are statistically significant. | Inflexibility: once it has started, the initial study design must remain unchanged throughout data collection. |
| Possibility of administration from remote locations using mail, email or telephone. | Survey questions tend to be close-ended and pre-empt and anticipate respondents' answers, leaving little space for elaborate and reflective responses from research participants. |
| Several questions may be asked about a topic. | |
| Initial flexibility in deciding how the questions will be administered. Various forms of administration are possible: namely, face-to-face interviews, telephone interviews, group questionnaires, written or oral surveys, or by electronic means. | High response rates must be secured but are not guaranteed. |
| | Participants may fail to recall information or to tell the truth. |
| High reliability: standardised questions make measurement more precise by enforcing uniform definitions upon participants. | Lack of contextualisation of responses. |
| Group comparisons: standardisation allows for the collection of similar data that can then be used to make comparisons between groups. | |
| High reliability: respondent subjectivity is greatly eliminated. | |

*Source:* http://writing.colostate.edu/guides/research/survey/com2d1.cfm

by David Farrington, was undertaken to test several hypotheses about delinquent trajectories. The investigators examined various issues, including: socioeconomic conditions, schooling, friendship, parent–child relationships, extracurricular activities, school records and criminal records.

According to Tonry *et al.* (1991), only longitudinal surveys provide information on cumulative phenomena and sequential patterns of behaviour and are able to investigate stability and continuity over time. An alleged strength of longitudinal designs is the possibility of prediction. It is claimed that longitudinal surveys are superior to cross-sectional studies in establishing an order of events. On the other hand, cross-sectional studies involve studying different groups of participants that share some given criteria (e.g. age or gender) at the same point in time. They can be likened to snapshots that depict adolescents and their attributes and past experiences at single moments. Like snapshots, cross-sectional studies can describe things and permit observers to know what is correlated with what, but they cannot tell us reliably what *precedes* what. The ESPAD survey is an example of a cross-sectional study. It tries to establish relationships between age of first use of a particular substance and patterns of use, and between leisure participation and substance use, among different cohorts of same-age students at different points in time. A longitudinal study, by contrast, would entail research with the same cohort over different time intervals. It could be likened to an unwinding videotape that shows, for example, whether children who struggle academically in school are more likely to hold positive attitudes towards substances or to use substances, or whether some children follow one developmental path while others follow another. Long-term longitudinal studies have one serious disadvantage: because they are conducted over a long period of time, attrition rates (loss of participants) are high (Tonry *et al.* 1991).

The longitudinal design provides the most accurate information about the continuity or discontinuity of behaviour through time and allows for the individual tracking of patterns of behaviour, as well as trends of development, within a particular cohort (group). However, it is costly and time consuming to study a large group of individuals over an extensive time span. Participants may, for various reasons, drop out of the study. Moreover, they may, through repeated administration of the same instrument (a questionnaire, for example), become too knowledgeable about it and consequently bias the results. Cross-sectional studies are more economical since they do not require the researcher to follow the development of each individual. In such studies, the evidence of change is inferred from differences between the groups involved in the study.

## Practice-based task 6.3  Longitudinal studies

Design a longitudinal study to explore changes in leisure patterns as adolescents progress through to emerging adulthood. Consider practical and logistical issues of engaging in a longitudinal study in your youth work context. Quickly list all the benefits you can of conducting longitudinal research with a group of participants on a set topic over a number of years. What challenges might you face in conducting such research?

## Box 6.2  Read more

*Methods of Studying Children: Longitudinal versus Cross-sectional Studies.* http://social.jrank.org/pages/411/Methods-Studying-Children-Longitudinal-versus-Cross-Sectional-Studies.html#ixzz0ayXn0rTt.

# Practical issues for the survey method

As a youth researcher-practitioner, you will need to make a series of decisions that are almost always present when undertaking social research. These relate to:

- population and sampling issues;
- administering the questionnaire;
- ethical issues.

## *Population and sampling*

In survey research a population refers to all the existing members of any given group. Since the population will normally be too large for each individual within it to be investigated, we would normally work with a representative sample from it. Depending on your practice context and subject area, negotiating access to a research population may well be the most problematic issue in youth practitioner-led research, and the youth researcher should consider how accessible a population is before embarking on any research project. Because of their active involvement in youth work practice, youth researchers may have access to groups of young people that are not accessible to other researchers: for example, in youth clubs or schools.

However, some groups, for example young sex workers or homeless youth may be particularly hard-to-reach. In the case of such research participants, a complete list of all the individuals belonging to the population is unavailable. This also has implications for representativeness. If one wishes to conduct a survey amongst young sex workers, working with a group accessing a service will not guarantee representation as it is unlikely that most sex workers would be accessing a service. Similarly, drug or alcohol users in treatment cannot be considered representative of users generally. The same would stand for young offenders in prison, or the homeless or domestic violence survivors utilising a shelter. If one is studying rates of school attendance and motivations for truancy, one is most likely to miss really truanting students if one conducts the research wholly in schools. Yet, the convenience of using captive audiences – or *convenience samples* – often leads youth researchers to use such samples despite their obvious limitations. In some circumstances the researcher may have little choice. For example, when studying populations engaged in high-risk behaviours, this choice should be dictated by concern for personal safety. Moreover, there may be protection issues (particularly when dealing with minors) that make accessing a population problematic. Youth workers may also want to reflect on the ethical dimensions of such decisions.

The hallmark of survey research is the concern with representativeness, and researchers have explored various methods for securing representative samples. Techniques referred to as probability sampling methods (explored below) do this well (e.g. Henry 1990; Kish 1965) and are the preferred sampling methods in survey research.

A probability sample is a *representative* subset of an entire population of people, events or variables. For example, if one were undertaking a study of university students' attitudes towards the EU policy on illegal immigration, the researcher would need to ensure that all university students from each faculty could be consulted in the study. In order to achieve a representative sample of a population, sampling must be done randomly. Probability sampling may be undertaken by a variety of techniques. The principal characteristics of some central sampling methodologies used in survey research are described below.

### Simple and systematic random sampling

Simple random sampling involves the selection of individuals to be surveyed from a list of the people in a population. Here every unit has an equal probability of occurring in the selected group; or, as Schofield (1996: 30) eloquently puts it, 'Random sampling means that every element in the population of interest has an *equal and independent* chance of being chosen.' As Schofield emphasises in simple random sampling, 'random' does not imply 'haphazard', and it is far from easy to achieve. To ensure precision, 'random number tables' or 'computerized number generators' are often used (Schofield 1996: 31), where numbers assigned to each unit (person in the population, for example) are selected randomly.

A variation of the simple random sample is the systematic selection procedure. This requires a list of all the people in the population. A random number is then assigned to each person interviewed: for example, selecting every tenth person in a particular list.

Despite their advantages, simple random sampling and systematic sampling share two significant disadvantages. First, they require a list of the entire population of interest so that random or systematic selection can be made. This is impossible, for example, in countries where there are no lists of all residents or citizens, and no one could personally afford to compile such a list. Second, it could be too expensive to interview a sample of a large sampling frame (the list of all those in the population being studied). Moreover, in the case of a systematic sample, we need to guard against *systematic bias*. Schofield (1996: 31) illustrates this as follows: 'for example, if the names in a school class were listed systematically as "boy, girl, boy, girl . . ." and we sampled every second name, we should obtain a sample made up of a single gender from a class made up of both genders in equal proportions'. This form of bias may be avoided by choosing what Schofield termsa 'suitable sampling interval', by which is meant the time or number elapsing between samples.

### Stratified random sampling

This technique is often used to overcome the problems mentioned above. Stratifying the sample means dividing the population into small, manageable chunks – or *strata* – and randomly sampling from each chunk. For example, in an opinion poll among young people to test their voting preferences prior to an election, it would be useful to break down one's sampling frame into different regions and then select samples from each region so that the final sample will be proportionate to the regional distribution of voters. In such instances, one would ensure that stratification reflects the characteristics of the population under scrutiny.

## Clustered sampling

Here the sample is based on a particular cluster – for example, all young voters from a particular geographic region – and then selecting one's sample from the identified cluster. Accuracy declines in cluster sampling. People who live in the same region may share similar voting preferences. Thus, recruiting participants from the same cluster yields less valid data than would be gained by taking into account different geographical regions.

## Quota sampling

Inaccurate findings are often attributed to the failure to employ such sampling techniques (e.g. Laumann *et al.* 1994). For example, some survey professionals often use a *quota sampling* method. This is a form of non-probability sampling, where after the sampling frame is divided into various sub-groups or strata, 'quotas of the desired number of cases are then calculated proportionally to the number of elements in these subgroups. These quotas are then divided up among the interviewers, who simply set out to find individuals who fit the required quota criteria' (Schofield 1996: 36). Although this method further minimises costs and may have 'intuitive appeal' to survey researchers, its main shortcoming is that it does not include any attempt at randomisation and hence makes establishing sample error an impossible task. As Schutt (1999: 130) contends, it is crucial for the researcher to be aware of the characteristics of a whole population to establish the appropriate quotas. This is often difficult to achieve.

Therefore, it is generally stressed that representative and probability sampling methods are essential to permit confident generalisation of results. This is difficult to achieve in non-probability sampling methods, such as theoretical or convenience sampling methods, defined by Patton (2001: 238) as the process of selecting 'incidents, slices of life, time periods, or people on the basis of their potential manifestation or representation of important theoretical constructs'. For a more detailed explanation of sampling techniques, Bryman (2008) provides an accessible guide.

**Table 6.2 Survey sampling methods: strengths and limitations**

| Sample type | Strengths | Limitations |
| --- | --- | --- |
| Simple and systematic random sampling | Does not require information about the sample population before sampling. | May be too cumbersome and impractical to use when large samples need to be generated. |
| | Relatively simple to undertake when a large sample is not required. | Less useful when sampling from regular and structured lists of elements. |
| | Sampling biases can be predetermined. | In instances where systematic random sampling is used, systematic bias may be introduced. |

## Table 6.2  continued

| Sample type | Strengths | Limitations |
| --- | --- | --- |
| Stratified sampling | More precise than random sampling, and not necessarily more costly.<br><br>Less risk of inadequate population sub-group representation.<br><br>Facilitates estimation and control of sampling error. | Researchers have to be especially vigilant in deciding which strata/variables to use in the process of sample selection as this can affect data interpretation negatively due to the over-representation of some population groups over others.<br><br>Requires a priori information on a population to be effective (e.g. electoral registers and so forth).<br><br>Accessibility to such listing can prove problematic and costly. |
| Cluster sampling | Further reduces costs.<br><br>Advantageous where sample population lists are unavailable or, if available, are inaccurate.<br><br>Useful in instances where populations are spread over large distances or time intervals.<br><br>Still includes elements of randomisation in contrast to non-probability methods, such as quota sampling. | Increases risk of sampling error.<br><br>Less efficient than random sampling methods and stratified sampling. |
| Quota sampling | Reduces costs and is relatively easy to administer.<br><br>Attuned to the 'intuitive appeal' of researchers (Schofield 1996: 36).<br><br>Can prove crucial in instances where data collection is needed quickly.<br><br>Useful for studies where randomisation is impossible or where the research topic | Participant selection necessitates and entails considerable interviewer/ fieldworker discretion, leading to different sources of sample bias.<br><br>Probability and randomness in sample selection are compromised.<br><br>Estimation and control of sampling error is difficult |

| Sample type | Strengths | Limitations |
|---|---|---|
| | does not concern a large amount of people. | (although sample errors in quotas are no greater than for a random sample). |
| | | Requires vigilance and control of fieldworkers/ interviewers to ensure that research participants are chosen on the basis of relevant criteria. |

*Sources:* Schofield 1996; Schutt 1999

In even the best surveys, there are inevitable biases in the demographic and attitudinal composition of samples obtained. Brehm (1993) writes how certain demographic groups are routinely represented in misleading numbers. Young and old adults, males, and people with the highest income levels are underrepresented, whereas people with the lowest education levels are overrepresented. Cialdini *et al.* (1992) found that people who agreed to be interviewed displayed particular characteristics, such as being socially responsible, possessing an internal locus of control and having high subjective well-being. This study showed that attitudes towards surveys, perceived survey participation of acquaintances and one's valuation of privacy are important factors that influence one's likelihood to participate in a survey. It may be thought that the higher the response rate, the less bias. But it is not necessarily true that representativeness increases automatically with increasing response rate. For example, Visser *et al.* (1996) examined self-administered mail and telephone surveys and showed that those with very low response rates can be more accurate than those with much higher response rates.

It is important to recognise the inherent limitations of non-probability sampling methods (such as theoretical or purposive sampling) and to draw conclusions about populations or differences between populations tentatively when non-probability sampling methods are used. But when probability sampling methods are used, it is no longer sensible to presume that lower response rates necessarily signal lower representativeness.

## Administering the survey

When administering a survey, steps must be taken to ensure as strong a response rate as possible. Large sample sizes are advised despite the fact that many types of survey, for example mail and telephone surveys, often have low response rates. Questionnaires may be distributed by mail, including a self-addressed envelope ready stamped for return posting. Mailed, self-administered surveys generally have low response rates. Schutt (1999: 254) holds that response rates in mailed surveys are unlikely to be any higher than 80 per cent and 'almost surely will be below 70 per cent unless procedures to maximize the response rate are followed to the letter'.

According to Schutt, procedures to encourage response rates may include using visuals to guide respondents, using simple and straightforward language in individual questions, limiting the number of open-ended questions in the questionnaire, using financial incentives and credible sponsors for the study, ensuring as eye-catching a design for the questionnaire as possible and, above all, contacting initial non-respondents through follow-up correspondence. The latter is known to encourage better response rates (Schutt 1999: 256).

A variant of the mailed survey is the household drop-off survey. This involves the researcher going to the person's home, business or any other setting and handing over the survey. The person is asked to mail it back or the researcher might offer to return to pick it up.

Other options for administering the questionnaire are face-to-face interviews or group surveys. Surveys conducted by interviews are far more personal than other survey forms and various ethical issues arise (anonymity and confidentiality, especially). In the personal interview, the interviewer works directly with the respondent. Unlike mail surveys, the interviewer has the opportunity to probe or ask follow-up questions. Interviews can be very time consuming and they are resource intensive, but group-administered questionnaires may avoid these problems because large numbers of people hand in their questionnaires simultaneously. In the group-administered questionnaire, a sample of respondents is brought together. The group questionnaire is very convenient and ensures a high response rate. If the respondents are unclear about the meaning of a question they can ask for clarification. In group administered surveys researchers should guard against participants feeling coerced to participate (Schutt 1999: 257). Such an eventuality may lead research participants to respond in ways they think the researcher requires.

Another accepted method for conducting surveys is by telephone (Schutt 1999). An inability to reach the sampled units and a tendency for a weak response rate, however, tend to affect the validity of this survey method. Brehm (1993) documents how telephone surveys rarely achieve response rates higher than 60 per cent. These and other limitations may be overcome by multiple call-backs, using carefully designed instructions for administering the survey and trying to ensure respondent focus and attention as much as possible (Schutt 1999: 257–262). Table 6.3 charts the strengths and weaknesses of different modes of survey administration.

In order to ensure as robust a research instrument as possible, a number of safeguards must be taken into account. Inappropriate wording and improper placement of questions within a survey questionnaire may yield biased results, thus affecting generalisability. Questions must be clearly and unambiguously set up. Double-barrelled or run-on questions must be avoided and questions should be worded to allow accurate transmission of respondents' answers to researchers. Loaded or biased words and terms can affect the reliability of the resulting data: for example, 'In your free time, would you *rather* read a book or *just* watch television?' Leading questions – that is, questions that suggest a certain response either literally or by implication, or contain a hidden premise – also require rigorous scrutiny and need to be weeded out: for example, 'Like most English young people, do you watch the popular soap *EastEnders* every Friday?' Questions that ask for highly detailed information and strong recollection should also be avoided: for example, 'In the past year, how many hours of television have you viewed with your family?' (Schutt 1999: 239–251).

### Table 6.3 Modes of survey administration

| Data collection method | Strengths | Limitations |
| --- | --- | --- |
| Street interviews | Suitable for short, structured interviews. Ideal for locating a general sample. | Not appropriate for lengthy interviews or those involving many questions.<br><br>Location of sub-groups is difficult.<br><br>Not ideal for open-ended questions. |
| Telephone | Very economic. Relatively efficient.<br><br>Possibility of reaching difficult samples. | Not everyone has a telephone.<br><br>Difficult to show stimulus material – unless sent through post previously.<br><br>Interview length is limited.<br><br>Increasing number of ex-directory/solus mobile usage. |
| Postal | Generally inexpensive.<br><br>Possibility of long questionnaires.<br><br>Respondents can take their time to consider their responses. | Poor response rates.<br><br>Non-representative samples. |
| In home | Appropriate environment for interview.<br><br>Face to face.<br><br>Able to show stimulus material.<br><br>Pre-recruitment of sample. | Expensive.<br><br>Time-consuming.<br><br>Respondent reluctance. |
| Internet | Economical.<br><br>Efficient.<br><br>Large sample sizes.<br><br>Minimum hassle 'all in one' software: e.g. Survey Monkey.<br><br>Visual material. | Not everyone has internet.<br><br>Low response rates. |

In the case of self-administered questionnaires, we must acknowledge that participants are required to be literate in the language of the researcher. Once again, with certain youth groups, this may pose a problem. Many researchers might take literacy among young people for granted, even though adult and youth illiteracy remains alarmingly high in Europe. The nature of the language utilised in the research tool is also important because, although respondents may have basic literacy skills, they may not be able to negotiate a technical questionnaire or one that is beyond their reading level. The age of the respondents is also an important issue: questionnaires aimed at young adolescents should be formatted in child friendly language. When conducting research with refugees, language can be a major stumbling block. While one always has the option to translate the questionnaires, it is important that meanings are not 'lost in translation'. The researcher must also be confident that important connotations in the research instrument are not culturally specific.

In times of economic recession, budgets for youth projects and research are becoming increasingly vulnerable, so the cost effectiveness of research remains an important consideration. Surveys are a relatively inexpensive option, especially if they are self-administered, as they can be easily administered from remote locations using mail, telephone and increasingly email. Survey Monkey is a potent tool because you can quickly create and administer a survey questionnaire with only basic computer literacy skills. Using this online tool, you can provide a link to your survey in an email or on your website, and respondents can submit their responses anonymously.

## Ethical issues

As already discussed in earlier chapters, ethical dilemmas constitute an important aspect of conducting research with young people. Three dimensions of ethics identified by Guillemin and Gillam (2004) may be considered in relation to practitioner-led quantitative youth research. *Procedural ethics* refers to the procedures of gaining ethical approval from the relevant boards and committees of the organisation or institution in which the youth researcher is working. *Ethics in practice* refers to the ethical issues that emerge as part of the research process, including the treatment of research participants, informed consent, coercion, privacy and deception. The issue of power and adult authority is also central and is highlighted by Best (2007) in her text on methodological issues in critical youth studies. Research with young people involves what has been termed 'studying down' (Best 2007: 12). Power is present at every stage of the research process: from when the research agenda is being articulated, in the data collection and in the analysis. Best (2007: 12) writes: 'An acknowledgment of the imbalance of power in research requires careful attention to the ways our methods, our definitional boundaries and our claims making construct a world and the groups in it as much as they express it.' The third dimension of research ethics relates to *accuracy*. It is essential that the researcher is factual in his/her reporting of findings.

In the UK, the Economic and Social Research Council (ESRC) has developed a Research Ethics Framework intended to sustain and encourage good ethical practice in UK social science research. There are *six* key principles of ethical research that the

ESRC expects to be followed. These provide a good framework for youth practitioner/researchers working within the quantitative tradition.

1   *Research should be designed, reviewed and undertaken to ensure integrity and quality.* Ethical research is methodologically sound research. Flaws in the research design or poorly developed research questions may contribute to results that are inaccurate and do not truly reflect the reality of the life word of young people. Policy and practice decisions are then taken on the basis of that research. The choice of research questions is also an ethical issue. Sackett (1979) identifies eight possible sites of bias in the research process: planning, design, data collection, data processing, data analysis, presentation, interpretation and publication. Altman (1980) emphasises that there is greatest need for expertise in the design stage because, although analysis or interpretation errors may be rectified, deficiencies in design are almost impossible to remedy. In the design stage, the researcher-practitioner should primarily look out for potential problems in sampling (considering those who are eligible to participate) and randomisation. The quantification of the phenomena under scrutiny is very important and variables need to be clearly defined and methods of measurement (reliability and validity) considered. The data collection, processing and analysis stages also present challenges. Jones (2000: 152) stresses that 'picking and choosing data just to make the results look better is unethical'. Incorrectly analysing data and using the wrong statistical tests in order to 'exaggerate the accuracy or explanatory power of the data' is similarly unethical. The choice of which data to analyse raises ethical questions and the presentation of results is open to unethical practice (for example, quoting the standard error of the mean as a measure of variability rather than variance because it is smaller). The interpretation of data is open to bias, as when associations are interpreted as causal relationships. The term 'significant' is also often misused.

2   *Informed consent.* In quantitative studies the information provided to respondents should clearly indicate the purpose of the research; how the research is being done; the uses to which the research will be put; and any possible risks to participants arising from participation. Researchers need to construct an information sheet documenting all of the above. This should be written in a user-friendly manner and in a language that research participants will be able to comprehend. In the case of an anonymous questionnaire used as the research tool for the survey, written consent may be waived (participation implies consent), but participants still need to be given the information that will enable them to make the decision to participate or not. In the case of minors consent must be sought not only from the participants themselves but from their parents/legal guardians.

3   *The confidentiality of information supplied by research subjects and the anonymity of respondents must be respected.* Surveys are by their nature often anonymous. However, collection procedures need to ensure that respondents feel secure that their identity is protected. The questionnaire must not include information that may identify particular individuals. In storage, researchers must take all steps to protect data. Research information stored on hard drives should be erased if the computer changes hands. In communicating research findings, care must be taken to respect

any undertakings of confidentiality given to respondents and to use a level of anonymity that protects the interests not only of the respondent but of the organisation they work for or with which they are otherwise involved. This can require fine judgement. To contextualise the research adequately, it may be necessary, or at least desirable, to provide information that could allow particular respondents or organisations to be identified, even if they are not named directly. Judgements of this kind need to be discussed with supervisors and more senior researchers, and may even need to be taken to an ethics committee.

4   *Research participants must participate voluntarily, free from any coercion.* Researchers should be aware that coercion might be introduced inadvertently. This is a particularly thorny issue when conducting research with young people who may have less power in relation to the researchers. Coercion may be subtle: for example, in the case of youth researchers conducting an evaluation in their own youth group or youth centre. Young people may feel that they may be discriminated against if they do not cooperate with the researchers in these situations.

5   *Harm to research participants must be avoided.* All research should be undertaken under the basic principle that it does not cause harm, allow harm to be inflicted, or otherwise damage the interests of any involved parties. Harm may be physical or psychological, or may result as a consequence of the information divulged. The potential for harm is stronger in research involving vulnerable groups or sensitive topics.

6   *The independence of research must be clear, and any conflicts of interest or partiality must be explicit.* It is paramount that social science researchers remain independent from the interests of stakeholders in executing a research study. Youth practitioners undertaking an evaluation study of a service provision they are engaged in should guard against any conflict of interest or partiality that may arise from their involvement in the study.

## Summary points

Brooker and Macpherson (1999) contend that practitioner research can become useful only when the research is informed by social science research principles. Nowhere is this more evident than with quantitative methods. This chapter has suggested how practitioner-researchers may ensure that sound precepts and practices inform their research efforts. Changes in the world of work – towards 'a reflexive learning society' and an increase in reflective practice – encourage practitioner research (Jarvis 1999). However, practitioner research will be taken seriously only if practitioner-researchers can be seen to have the requisite skills to conduct proper research that satisfies the rigorous requirements of the social science community. Many practitioner-researchers might think that scientific research methods are boring, irrelevant and difficult to grasp. Still, many of the concepts applied in scientific research are already well known to the novice researcher in an informal manner. This chapter has helped to formalise and clarify core ideas that have been gathered through everyday experience and practice as well as problematise taken-for-granted ideas.

Case study 6.1

Exploring drug and alcohol use among
young people in Europe

Drug and alcohol use has become a major concern in public policy generally and youth policy in particular. The ESPAD (European School Project on Alcohol and Other Drugs) documents adolescent substance use in Europe from a comparative perspective and utilises the survey approach, collecting data on the use of substances among fifteen- and sixteen-year-olds attending school in Europe in a comparable and standardised manner. All participating countries utilise the same standardised quantitative survey tool.

The ESPAD survey takes place every four years and allows youth researchers to monitor the trends of adolescent substance use in European countries and to compare national trends. It seeks to identify changes in youth drug use in specific countries, to understand the context of adolescent drug use, its predictors and consequences and therefore serves as an important resource for policy-makers. Effective strategies may be implemented in order to prevent or halt the development of addictive careers. Data generated by the ESPAD survey, when analysed together with other information on drugs and alcohol use, allows youth researchers to understand the extent and patterns of use and concurrent beliefs, attitudes and behaviours. The statistical nature of the project and the fact that the survey questionnaire contains questions regarding demographics allow for the analysis of data in accordance with subgroups. This comprehensive picture of adolescent substance use can also alter misconceptions about this commonly stereotyped sector of the population.

This case study provides readers with a practical example of how the issues discussed in this chapter are addressed in real life research. We will show how population and sampling, field procedure, reliability, validity, anonymity and test construction, including language, are addressed. It provides an exemplar for the use of the survey method in youth and community studies.

## Research design: a standardised survey

### The ESPAD research tool

The ESPAD study benefits from a standardised research tool. Since the ESPAD survey collects data to support the comparison of trends across different countries in Europe, a standardised tool is used. The survey tool is an anonymous questionnaire that takes an average of fifty minutes to complete. It includes questions about socio-demographic characteristics and alcohol-, tobacco- and drug-related variables. It also contains questions measuring beliefs and attitudes.

Adjustments are made to some questions to make them relevant to the cultural context in which the questionnaire is being administered. The principal language of the country where the questionnaire is being administered is used.

## Population and sampling

The target population for the ESPAD survey comprises students who are or will become sixteen years old during the year of data collection (Hibell *et al.* 2004). It is recommended that each national net sample comprises 2,400 students. Cluster sampling is used and is based on whole school classes as the final sampling units (Bjarnason and Morgan 2002). This procedure is more economical than sampling individual students and also increases respondents' perceptions of anonymity. Sampling individual students and asking them to fill out a questionnaire individually might influence the truthfulness of their answers and therefore bias the results of the study.

## Field procedure

The time period for the administration of the research tool is also standardised across countries. March/April is the recommended period of data collection. It is up to each ESPAD research team to decide whether teachers or research assistants carry out the survey. Survey leaders receive written instructions describing how to perform the survey and how to fill out the standardised classroom report. The questionnaires are answered anonymously and individual envelopes are provided for the students to seal the completed forms, making respondents feel safe and anonymous. To avoid discussions of the survey among the students, data collection is done at the same time in case several classes are sampled from the same school.

## Reliability

Reliability, as discussed earlier in the chapter, is the extent to which repeated measurements used under the same conditions produce the same results. Before embarking on data collection, the ESPAD research tool was tested for reliability at the commencement of the project utilising data from different questions within the ESPAD questionnaire. More specifically, one measure of reliability involved measuring the inconsistency between two sets of questions measuring lifetime prevalence for different drugs. 'The other measure was a quotient between the proportion of students who on the "honesty question" answered that they "already said" that they had used cannabis and the proportion who actually gave this answer' (http://www.drugslibrary.stir.ac.uk/documents/espad student2007.pdf).

Test–retest is perhaps the most effective way of measuring reliability. Test–retest reliability is measured by administering the same test to the same sample on two different occasions. If there is no substantial change in the construct being measured between the two occasions then the tool is reliable. However, in the ESPAD pilot study it was not possible to do a test–retest study at *the individual level* since the respondents needed to remain completely anonymous. Therefore, *different students* in seven countries were asked to complete the questionnaire on their use of alcohol and drugs on two separate occasions with a delay period of three–five days (Hibell *et al.* 2000). No significant differences in the consumption patterns were found between the two data collections in any of the countries. This was true for alcohol consumption as well as for drug prevalence, which suggests that reliability was high in the pilot study.

## Validity

The validity of collected data is a major concern in all surveys, and especially in relation to sensitive behaviours, like drug use. High reliability is a necessary but insufficient condition for validity. In the ESPAD study, validity is the degree to which the ESPAD questionnaire measures aspects of students' *actual* consumption. The primary condition for obtaining any valid data in a survey is that respondents actually receive the questionnaire and are willing to complete it. For ethical reasons, participation in any study must be voluntary. For ESPAD, few students were reported to have refused participation. Issues such as the time given to complete the questionnaire, the comprehension of the questions, willingness to answer honestly and understanding of the questions may also affect validity. Students must also be willing to answer the questions.

## Anonymity

With surveys that measure involvement in illicit behaviour, such as drug use, an important issue influencing validity is that respondents answer honestly. This will be achieved only if it can be guaranteed that there will be no negative consequences once they have reported their behaviour. Anonymity is therefore a very important concern and is incorporated into the standardisation of the field procedure. After answering their questionnaires, participants in the ESPAD study are required to place their responses in a sealed envelope.

## Logical consistency

Logical consistency is crucial for the reliability of a study. ESPAD researchers use responses to questions related to the prevalence of lifetime drug use, drug use over the last year and the last month as measures of such consistency. For such measures to be consistent, the prevalence of drug use over the last year cannot exceed lifetime use and so forth.

## Construct validity

This refers to the extent to which variables are related to one another in a valid fashion. It is established by using existing theories, results from earlier studies and logical inference. Students who report a high use of different substances should also report that their friends use substances extensively.

## Language and the cultural context

The comparability of the ESPAD questionnaire across countries is vital, making translation an important aspect of validity. The standard ESPAD questionnaire is written in English. In non-English-speaking countries the questionnaire is translated back by another translator and the original and the back-translated versions are compared. The equivalency of questionnaires is a matter not only of literal translation but of equivalent understanding. Thus, the question should be 'understood' in the same way in all countries irrespective of the model questionnaire's original wording. Questions should be culturally adjusted to the country situation.

## Absent students

Naturally, a survey questionnaire can measure only the replies of those who are present to take it. In the case of school samples, youth researchers are aware that there are young people who are consistently absent and who may be more likely to be engaged in illicit behaviour than those who are attached and committed to education (Hirschi 1969). In the ESPAD context the alcohol and drug involvement among absent students can be seen as a major methodological problem.

*Source:* http://www.espad.org/documents/Espad/
ESPAD_reports/ESPAD_17-18_Year_Old_2003.pdf

# References

Ackoff, R.L. (1962) *Scientific method: optimising applied research decisions*, New York: John Wiley.

Altman, D.G. (1980) 'Statistics and ethics in medical research, VI: Presentation of results', *British Medical Journal*, 281: 1542–1544.

Attewell, P. and Rule, J. (1991) 'Survey and other methodologies applied to IT impact research: experiences from a comparative study of business computing', in K. Kraemer (ed.), *The information systems research challenge: survey research methods*, Volume 3, Boston, MA: Harvard Business School Press, 299–315.

Beniart, S., Anderson, B., Lee, S. and Utting, D. (2002) *A national survey of problem behaviour and associated risk and protective factors among young people*, York: Joseph Rowntree Foundation.

Best, A. (2007) *Representing youth: methodological issues in critical youth studies*, New York: New York University Press.

Bjarnason, T. and Morgan, M. (2002) *Guidelines for sampling procedures in the School Survey Project on Alcohol and Other Drugs*, Stockholm: Swedish Council for Information on Alcohol and Other Drugs.

Black, J. and Champion, D.J. (1976) *Methods and issues in social research*, New York: Wiley.

Brehm (1993) *The phantom respondents: opinion surveys and political representation*, Ann Arbor: University of Michigan Press.

Brooker, R. and Macpherson, I. (1998) 'Communicating the outcomes of practitioner research: an exercise in self-indulgence or a serious professional responsibility', paper presented at the Second International Practitioner Research Conference, Sydney, 9–11 July.

Brooker, R. and Macpherson, I. (1999) 'Communicating the processes and serious professional responsibility', *Educational Action Research*, 7 (2): 45–58.

Brown, S. ( 2005) *Understanding youth and crime*, Buckingham: Open University Press.

Bryman, A. (2008) *Social research methods*, Oxford: Oxford University Press.

Bulmer, M. (1982) 'The merits and demerits of covert participant observation', in M. Bulmer (ed.), *Social research ethics*, London: Macmillan, 217–251.

Chisholm, L. (2006) 'Youth research and the youth sector in Europe: perspectives, partnerships and promise', in M. Milmiester and H. Williamson (eds), *Dialogues and networks: organizing exchanges between youth field actors*, Luxembourg: Scientific – Editions PHI, 23–28.

Cialdini, R., Braver, S., Wolf, W. and Pitts, S. (1992) 'Who says no to legitimate survey requests? Evidence from a new method for studying the causes of survey non-response', paper presented at the Third International Workshop on Household Survey Nonresponse, The Hague, Netherlands, September.

Cicourel, A. ( 1964) *Method and measurement in sociology*, New York: Wiley.

Clark, M. (1999) 'The pursuit of a criminal career: a biographical approach', unpublished doctoral dissertation, University of Sheffield.

Coady, M. and Bloch, S. (1996) *Codes of ethics and the professions*, Melbourne: Melbourne University Press.

Coolican, H. (1990) *Research methods in psychology*, London: Hodder.

Creswell, J. (2003) *Research design: qualitative, quantitative, and mixed methods approaches*, 2nd edn, London: Sage.

Cronbach, L.J., Rajaratnam, N. and Gleser, G.C. (1963) 'Theory of generalizability: a liberalization of reliability theory', *British Journal of Statistical Psychology*, 16: 137–163.

Crotty, M. (1998) *Foundations of social research: meaning and perspective in the research process*, London: Sage.

ESRC, *Research ethics framework*. http://www.esrcsocietytoday.ac.uk/ESRCInfoCentre/Images/ESRC_Re_Ethics_Frame_tcm6-11291.pdf.

Foucault, M. (1975) *Discipline and punish: the birth of the prison*, New York: Random House.

Frankfort-Nachmias, C. and Nachmias, D. (1996) *Research methods in the social sciences*, 5th edn, London: Arnold.

Gable, G. (1994) 'Integrating case study and survey research methods: an example in information systems', *European Journal of Information Systems*, 3 (2): 112–126.

Graham, J. and Bowling, B. (1995) *Young people and crime*, Home Office Research Study No. 145, London: Home Office.

Guillemin, M. and Gillam, L. (2004) 'Ethics, reflexivity, and "ethically important moments" in research', *Qualitative Inquiry*, 10: 261–280.

Hargreaves, D. (1996) *Teaching as a research-based profession: possibilities and prospects*, London: Teacher Training Agency.

Hammersley, M. (1987) 'Some notes on the terms "validity" and "reliability"', *British Educational Research Journal*, 13 (1): 73–81.

Henry, G. (1990) *Practical sampling*, Newbury Park, CA: Sage.

Hibell, B., Andersson, B., Ahlström, S., Balakireva, O., Bjarnason, T., Kokkevi, A. and Morgan, M. (2000) *The ESPAD report 2003: alcohol and other drug use among students in 30 European countries*, Stockholm: CAN.

Hibell, B., Andersson, B., Bjarnason, T., Ahlström, S., Balakireva, O., Kokkevi, A. and Morgan, M. (2004) *The ESPAD report 2003: alcohol and other drug use among students in 35 European countries*, Stockholm: CAN.

Hirschi, T. (1969) *Causes of delinquency*. Berkeley: University of California Press.

Huitt, W. (1998) 'Critical thinking: an overview', *Educational Psychology Interactive*. http://www.edpsycinteractive.org/topics/cogsys/critthnk.html.

Jarvis, P. (1999) *The practitioner-researcher*, San Francisco: Jossey-Bass.

Jick, T. (1983) 'Mixing qualitative and quantitative methods: triangulation in action', in J. Van Maanen (ed.), *Qualitative methodology*, Beverly Hills, CA: Sage, 135–148.

Johnston, J.M. and Pennypacker, H.S. (1980) *Strategies and tactics of human behavioural research*, Hillsdale, NJ: Lawrence Erlbaum Associates.

Jones, A. (2000) 'Changing traditions of authorship', in A. Jones and F. Mclellan (eds), *Ethical issues in biomedical publication*, Baltimore, MD: Johns Hopkins University Press, 3–29.

Kaplan, B. and Duchon, D. (1988) 'Combining qualitative and quantitative methods in information systems research: a case study', *MIS Quarterly*, 12 (4): 571–586.

Kerlinger, F. (1964) *Foundations of behavioural research*, New York: Holt.

Kish, L. (1965) *Survey sampling*, New York: John Wiley and Sons.

Laumann, E., Gagnon, J., Michael, R. and Michaels, S. (1994) *The social organization of sexuality: sexual practice in the United States*, Chicago: University of Chicago Press.

Lehner, P. (1979) *Handbook of ethological methods*, New York: Garland, STPM Press.

Locke R. (1989) *Management and higher education since 1940*, New York: Cambridge University Press.

Patton, M. (2001) *Qualitative research and evaluation methods*, 2nd edn, Thousand Oaks, CA: Sage.

Punch, K. (2005) *Introduction to social research: quantitative and qualitative approaches*, London: Sage.

Raby, R. (2007) 'Children in sex, adults in crime: constructing and confining teens', *Resources for Feminist Research/Documentation sur la recherche feministe*, 31 (3/4): 9–28.

Robinson, G. (1998) *Methods and techniques in human geography*, London: Hodder.

Sackett, D.L. (1979) 'Bias in analytic research', *Journal of Chronic Diseases*, 32: 51–63.

Schofield, W. (1996) 'Survey sampling', in R. Sapsford and V. Jupp (eds), *Data collection and analysis*, London: Sage, 25–55.

Schutt, R. (1999) *Investigating the social world: the process and practice of research*, Thousand Oaks, CA: Pine Forge Press.

Schutz, A. (1976) *Collected papers*, Volume 2: *Studies in social theory*, The Hague: Martinus Nijhoff.

Swingewood, A. (2000) *A short history of sociological thought*, London: Palgrave Macmillan.

Tonry, M., Ohlin, L. and Farrington, D. (1991) *Human development and criminal behavior: new ways of advancing knowledge*, New York: Springer-Verlag.

Vidich, A. and Shapiro, G. (1955) 'A comparison of participant-observation and survey data', *American Sociological Review*, 20: 28–33.

Visser, P., Krosnick, J., Marquette, J. and Curtin, M. (1996) 'Mail surveys for election forecasting? An evaluation of the Columbus Dispatch Poll', *Public Opinion Quarterly*, 60: 181–227.

Wyn, R. and White, J. (2008) *Youth and society: exploring the social dynamics of youth experience*, Oxford: Oxford University Press.

## Internet sources

http://home.ubalt.edu/ntsbarsh/Business-stat/opre504.htm

http://rds.homeoffice.gov.uk/rds/pdfs/r127.pdf

http://social.jrank.org/pages/411/Methods-Studying-Children-Longitudinal-versus-Cross-Sectional-Studies.html#ixzz0ayXn0rTt

http://writing.colostate.edu/guides/research/survey/com2d1.cfm

http://www.education.gov.uk/rsgateway/DB/SFR/s000619/index.shtml

http://www.eryica.org/files/Expertmeeting%20Youthwork%20March2010%20PreAnnouncement.pdf

http://www.jrf.org.uk/publications/national-survey-problem-behaviour-and-associated-risk-and-protective-factors-among-young

http://www.espad.org/

http://www.esrc.ac.uk/esrcinfocentre/images/esrc_re_ethics_frame_tcm6-11291.pdf

http://www.library.carleton.ca/ssdata/surveys/doc/pdf_files/csdd-uk-61-81-cbk.pdf

http://www.un.org/esa/socdev/rwss/docs/2003/chapter2.pdf

# 7 Documentary research and secondary data

John Barker and Pam Alldred

## Overview

Youth practitioners work in organisations that document and count numerous aspects of social life. Our day-to-day professional lives require us to digest and implement policy documents, reports and guidelines, to contribute to numerous information-gathering exercises, to complete end-of-project evaluations and to ask service users to complete survey forms. The amount and types of documenting and counting are arguably multiplying with the intensifying demands of accountability. Researchers can also use data that is collected through organisations' everyday practices, often in dramatically distinct ways, to allow new critical insights into the social functions of organisations and wider sociological problems.

This chapter provides a critical introduction to documents and secondary data, exploring how such collections of documents and data can be used for research. It explains what sources might be used, what types of analysis might be conducted and what secondary research might achieve. Included are some pointers and tips that we hope will help youth practitioners to undertake this type of research, perhaps for the first time.

## Definitions

Many societies, cultures and organisations count and document, including recording individuals' events (such as birth, achievement, marriage and death) and organisations' records of client use and feedback. Indeed, gathering and generating information is central to the contemporary modern age, since, as Atkinson and Coffey (2004: 5) argue,

> a quintessentially modern kind of social formation is thoroughly dependent on paperwork. Administrators, accountants, lawyers, civil servants, managers at all levels, and other experts or specialist functionaries [and youth practitioners, we might add] are all routinely, often extensively, involved in the production and

consumption of written records and other kinds of document. If we wish to under-stand how such organisations [or societies] work and how people work with/in them, we cannot afford to ignore their various activities as readers and writers.

However, although documents and data are pervasive throughout many contemporary settings where we might want to conduct research (McCulloch 2004), they are often overlooked as sources of data. In fact, counting and documenting generate data that can be used for social research in different ways. Much youth work-related documen-tation, such as service user profiles, client contact figures and patterns, and indicators of local issues or of outcomes, can have another life in the realm of social research. These offer insights into events, the ideas or intentions behind them or how they were expe-rienced. May (2001: 176) refers to documents as 'the sedimentation of social practices'. Analysing them can generate understanding of something that is otherwise too 'every-day' to seem worthy of analysis, so fundamental it usually escapes scrutiny, or about which there are strong values, taboos or assumptions. Scrutinising outcome indicators in documentary evidence can be insightful in highlighting the kinds of 'knowledges' that are deemed important and legible within particular policy/practice contexts. For instance, figures indicating the degree to which teenage pregnancy is considered a 'prob-lem' in a given area may have implications for funding and reputation, but may tell us nothing of local meanings given to childbearing, either by the community (were these planned births to women who have married young and therefore socially approved?) or individually (what sense do individuals make of their reproductive and sexual experiences?). Secondary research also allows insight without changing the phenomenon being investigated. New data may not be necessary to develop insights and inform practice.

Before continuing, let us define our key terms.

## Secondary research

Whilst data collected by oneself (see Chapters 4, 5 and 6) produces primary data, secondary research is an investigation using evidence or data that have not been col-lected by the researcher but rather produced by someone else for another purpose (Clark 2005). Secondary research can take a wide variety of forms, including documentary research (using documents that were not produced with research in mind, such as accident report forms, session debrief notes, youth centre behaviour codes, or policy documents), and secondary data analysis – that is, the re-analysis of data collected in another research project. For example, Papasolomontos and Christie (1998) discuss how researchers from different academic disciplines have undertaken educational research conducting secondary analysis using national government surveys, such as the Youth Cohort Study.

## Documents

A very broad range of materials can be seen as documents. Every year, central government, local authorities and other organisations generate huge numbers of documents. In the UK, *Every Child Matters* (DCSF 2003), *Youth Matters* (DCSF 2005) and local authority-produced documents such as children's and young people's plans are easy-to-recognise examples of documents in the public domain. Other forms of official documents include birth, marriage and death certificates. Documents can also include organisations' internal papers (e.g. minutes of meetings and internal strategy papers). Youth practitioners may find it easier to access these since they work in organisations that generate, digest and respond to a wider number of public and policy documents. Your organisation may have its own policy documents (such as drugs policy, behaviour code, etc.), meeting minutes, annual reports and monitoring statistics, referral criteria, debrief forms, funding applications, project descriptions, job descriptions, publicity, posters, press releases and so on. More personal and private examples of documents include letters, memoirs and historical inventories.

Although we may initially consider documents as paper based, more recently our definition has expanded to include documents written and saved electronically or digitally. As we critically discuss later in the chapter, the internet has become a key (if often problematic) source of written texts (May 2001). Historical texts may be recorded on other materials (e.g. inscriptions on gravestones or prison walls can be seen as text). Furthermore, as Parker and the Bolton Discourse Network (1999) illustrate, a wide range of cultural phenomena (from toothpaste packets to radio phone-ins) can be rendered as text.

## Documentary research

Documentary research is the process by which these texts are used as the empirical data for research (May 2001). As documents help to construct how people see the world (they urge us to act, perform and talk in particular ways), they are useful sources of data for youth practitioners since they can tell us about relevant political frameworks and professional practices. They also tell us a great deal about priorities, agendas and the ways in which young people and youth are constructed. Documents also enable youth practitioners to explore historical as well as contemporary events. Exploring the history of specific phenomena (e.g. the development of a particular service for young people) provides valuable contextual background to understanding how contemporary services are shaped. Historical research also enables us to consider the constantly changing ways of conceptualising young people, youth work and youth services. Whilst classic studies remind us that the development of youth culture is relatively recent, a closer examination of policy documents illustrates the ebb and flow of different political priorities and how this has re-envisioned our work: for example, the radical agendas of the 1970s and 1980s, the influence of the UK Children Acts 1989 and 2004, the Children's Rights and Participation movements, and the UN Convention on the Rights of the Child. A historical approach also reminds us of the non-inevitability of youth services and how 'conventional wisdom' is often less certain or stable than we might think. Historical research tells us that in another time or place, the issues faced by young people may be very different and that we may have organised youth provision in radically different ways.

---

**Case study 7.1**

**An example of documentary research**

---

Elizabeth Gagen's (2000, 2004, 2006) work is an exciting example of documentary research exploring historical events. Her research considers the increasing focus on children's physical fitness, the development of public supervised playgrounds in the USA in the early years of the twentieth century and how these activities promoted patriotism and specific gender roles. Her research draws upon a manuscript collection, including annual reports of playgrounds, public information sheets, newspaper articles (*circa* 1900–1910), in addition to academic and non-academic books, pamphlets and photographs from the relevant era. As she vividly describes:

> In the New York Public Library a disordered box of loose photographs, catalogued as 'Photographs of New York City schools, circa 1900', provides a rare visual archive of school life at the turn of the 19th century. Among the images of school and playground life, of carefully ordered classrooms with individual desks in uniform ranks, curious callisthenic exercises performed in polished wooden gymnasia, and craft-work classes where girls stitch samplers and boys carve unidentifiable objects from hunks of wood there is a photograph of a science display. A small collection of specimen jars present the dissected guts of a frog and various other biological objects preserved in formaldehyde for the purposes of scientific observation. Alongside the 'Heart of Ox' and 'Intestines of Sheep', sits 'Brain of Child'.
>
> (Gagen 2006: 827)

Gagen's graphic descriptions of these exotic sources are intriguing and inspire us to want to know more. Photographs and quoted extracts are used as examples of data to illustrate the function of physical fitness in schools and playgrounds (for example, to reproduce gender-specific roles through gender-appropriate play activities). Gagen's analysis enables her to consider the different kinds of identities that are forged and promoted through playgrounds and leisure.

## Practice-based task 7.1  Uncovering documentary data

1   Following on from Case study 7.1, where might you look for similar documentary evidence to explore the history of young people, leisure and play in the UK?

2   Youth practitioners are ideally suited to accessing documentary materials as they work in organisations that may store documents. Does the organisation you work for have an archive of materials? It might not be called an archive – rather a storeroom where annual reports, strategy documents, leaflets and photographs are kept. 'Brain of Child' notwithstanding, what do you think might be held in this archive?

3   If your organisation has an accessible archive, spend some time looking through it. Hours can pass quickly as you become engrossed in reading fascinating documents. What strikes you as most interesting about these historical documents?

4   If there is no official archive, think about alternative, less formal sources of archiving. For example, ask the longest-standing person you know in your organisation what old documents (e.g. reports, leaflets, strategy documents) they have.

5   What do you think might be the value of these specific 'historical' documents you have found for contemporary youth policy and practice?

### Secondary data analysis

Secondary data generally refers to quantitative survey data (see Chapter 6) that has been collected for a particular purpose but is available for other researchers to reuse and analyse (White 2003). Vast amounts of data (such as census data or teenage pregnancy figures) are available for secondary analysis. These can offer youth practitioners the chance to explore issues in more depth, at a larger scale or in places that may not otherwise be accessible.

Choosing between different forms of secondary research does not just entail technical decisions about 'what works' or what is available but relates to methodological debates about how to generate knowledge (McCulloch 2004). Documentary, text-based research is typically (though not always) associated with qualitative approaches to research, those that focus on in-depth meanings and explorations of everyday phenomena (see Chapter 5). Secondary data analysis typically refers to a quantitative approach to research, focusing upon exploring large-scale trends through translating phenomena into numbers to consider statistical relationships. However, there may be overlap: we cannot neatly distinguish between qualitative text and quantitative datasets. Documentary research can involve quantification (as we discuss later, a content analysis may involve counting the number of times an item appears in a document); secondary data analysis may involve qualitative datasets (e.g. interview transcripts); and quantitative survey data may include qualitative responses to open-ended questions.

## Why do secondary research?

Three broad reasons can be given for conducting secondary research (Kitchin and Tate 2000). First, it might not be practically possible to collect primary data (Miller and Alvarado 2005). Secondary research enables us to conduct research without having to be present during a historical occasion (for example, by analysing what young political activists wrote in their diaries in 1968, or young people wrote in letters during the First World War). Second, secondary research allows researchers to explore existing data using a different form of analysis than previously conducted. For instance, given the greater openness about homosexuality today, we might re-analyse historical interviews to see what might be hinted at but could not be spoken explicitly. Third, youth practitioners who are simultaneously engaged in professional practice and study may not have the time or money to conduct primary research.

There are three broad ways in which secondary research can contribute to the research process. First, secondary research can illustrate the context for primary research, providing a description of the people, places, events or trends that we may then explore through primary research. It can help justify primary research (e.g. 'secondary research shows us that knife crime is a growing problem for young people in some inner-city locations'). Second, secondary research helps us to make comparisons. Collecting primary data replicating the methods of an existing study enables us to compare findings with the existing dataset to explore trends across time, different scales (e.g. comparing national trends with data collected in one local authority) or countries (White 2003). Third, rather than using secondary data in conjunction with primary data, it can form the entire body of evidence for research.

## Sources of secondary data

Secondary research can draw data from archives and deposits that offer quantitative or qualitative datasets, or hold documentary material. Key sources include the following:

1   *Government departments.* Governments collect a wealth of information on their citizens, including young people, generating vast numbers of secondary datasets. In the UK these include the ten-yearly census and other national statistics focusing on housing, crime, education, employment, health and morbidity. Government data are often seen as authoritative, robust and valid, although, as we discuss shortly, there are critiques of this (White 2003). Data are often available at a variety of scales. In addition to national and regional trends, some datasets in the UK are

available at ward level, and Super Output Areas look at units of 1,500 residents. Whilst some datasets provide snapshots of contemporary issues, longitudinal studies (conducted or repeated over a long period of time) and cohort studies (following a specific sample of individuals from, for example, birth or leaving school) provide opportunities to explore trends over time.

UK National Statistics (http://www.statistics.gov.uk) makes available UK-wide government datasets. Scotland has its own agency (http://www.gro-scotland.gov.uk/statistics/index.html), as do Northern Ireland (http://www.nisra.gov.uk/) and Wales (http://wales.gov.uk/topics/statistics/). These offer access to a vast number of datasets of interest to youth practitioners. Mainstream datasets focusing on employment, health, crime, housing, family and so on can be interrogated by age, so that it is possible to explore general trends (e.g. within the British Social Attitudes survey) specifically in relation to young people. A number of government data sources focus solely on the experiences of young people, including:

- *The Longitudinal Study of Young People in England (LSYPE)*. This began in 2004 and brings together data from several sources, including annual interviews with 21,000 young people and their families. To date, six rounds of interviews with each young person have been conducted, exploring key factors affecting educational progress and attainment and transitions after compulsory education.
- *The Youth Cohort Study (YCS)*. Since 1985, this longitudinal survey has explored 30,000 young people's education and labour market experiences, their training and qualifications. It contacts a sample of young people in the spring following the end of compulsory education, then interviews them annually, typically for three years.

2   *The Economic and Social Data Service* (http://www.esds.ac.uk/). This UK-based national data service run by the Universities of Essex and Manchester provides access to an extensive range of quantitative and qualitative data collected by academic research and government surveys. Its main types of data are:

- *ESDS Government* contains large-scale government surveys, such as the Labour Force Survey and the General Household Survey, and is an alternative site to access youth-focused datasets, such as the Youth Cohort Study.
- *ESDS Longitudinal* holds major UK surveys following individuals over time, such as the British Household Panel Survey.
- *ESDS Qualidata* provides a range of multimedia qualitative data sources.
- *ESDS International* offers multinational research data, such as the World Bank's World Development Indicators, and survey data. Again, mainstream datasets exploring all age ranges of the population can be analysed specifically for young people.

3   *The Public Records Office* (also known as the National Archive) is the UK government's official archive holding public documents and records dating back over

1,000 years. A wealth of government records, including court proceedings and maps, are available to download (http://www.nationalarchives.gov.uk/documents online/). Also available are family history records, including census and military service records (although individual births, marriages and deaths post-1837 are held at the General Register's Office and are available online through specialist organisations).

4    *International organisations.* A number of organisations collate and assemble international datasets to enable international secondary analysis. The Eurostat Information Service (http://epp.eurostat.ec.europa.eu/) provides data to enable comparisons between European Union member countries. Themes include the economy, transport and environment as well as population and social conditions. Much data can be analysed by age, so it is possible to explore trends relating to young people. Specific youth-focused datasets include youth transitions from education to employment and post-compulsory education participation rates. UNICEF's Child Info website (http://www.childinfo.org/) measures the situation of children (and women) across the world through the collection and analysis of data (available for download) on a number of themes, including child survival and development, education and gender equality, child protection and HIV/AIDS. International datasets raise challenges for secondary research. Directly comparing statistics from individual countries can be complex, as definitions vary (for example, the ages encompassed under the term 'young people' differ widely). Processes of data collection may also vary (e.g. literacy rates may affect the validity of a self-completion questionnaire survey in parts of the world). Language may be another limitation, since ideas, concepts and words may not translate across different cultural contexts (Ansell *et al.* 2007).

5    *The media.* Newspaper archives are a valuable source of information about young people's lives, and at the local level can provide the history of a local youth centre or of youth-led campaigns. There is also a rapidly growing media industry produced for or by young people (e.g. the UK Youth Parliament's publications, magazines and programmes made by young people, and youth-based internet forums). However, increasingly one has to pay to view newspaper articles online. Articles are viewed out of context, divorced from the original newspaper location and without surrounding advertisements. Crucially, newspapers and other media must be treated with caution as secondary data sources since they are selective, written for particular audiences and their stories may be biased due to editorial steer, political perspective or errors (Macdonald 2008). Newspaper coverage often portrays young people in particular ways: for example, routinely generating 'moral panics' that pathologise young people's behaviour.

6    *Grey literature.* This term refers to literature or evidence created outside standard commercial, academic or state publishing and distribution channels. The internet contains a vast amount of grey literature, produced by lobbying groups, voluntary organisations, collectives, community groups and individuals. Respected organisations, such as the National Youth Agency and the National Society for the Prevention of Cruelty to Children (NSPCC), have websites containing documents or datasets of high quality. However, we must be cautious about the use of grey

literature in general. Such information is often unregulated, bypassing the routine control, editing and review processes to which other data are subject to ensure levels of quality, robustness and validity (Leveille and Chamberland 2010).

## Practice-based task 7.2  Downloading qualitative data

The Economic and Social Data Service (http://www.esds.ac.uk/) data archive holds much data of interest to youth practitioners. Registration is required to use the service. To download information, you need to complete a 'register of use of data' where you state how you want to use the materials.

1   Go online and register with ESDS (http://www.esds.ac.uk/)

2   Use the search engine to explore data of relevance to youth practitioners.

3   Undertake a search for 'young people and alcohol'. There are a large number of deposits – our search found 156 entries, ranging from the 'British Crime Survey' to 'Resisting Subjugation: Law and Power amongst the Santal of India and Bangladesh, 2002–2004'. Look for a specific qualitative dataset N 6217 'Branded Consumption and Social Identification: Young People and Alcohol Study, 2006–2007', led by Griffin and Szmigin. (If you cannot access this, find a similar deposit focusing on young people and alcohol.) 'Study description' provides contextual information, including that the qualitative dataset of 89 participants consists of 16 focus groups and 8 semi-structured individual interviews. The 'study description' page links to supplementary information pages. The 'data list' displays background socio-demographic information about participants. The 'user guide' provides documentary information relating to the original collection of the data (end-of-project report, letters of invitation, informed consent forms, interview schedules). Copies of the interview transcripts can be downloaded in compressed (zip) files.

4   Read a sample of the interview transcripts. Do you get a flavour of the interviews even though you were not present?

## Evaluating and assessing secondary sources

Having identified different sources, we need to think about how we might assess the potential value of secondary data. The following nine points explore ways to evaluate data sources critically:

1   *Secondary research as cultural product.* All secondary data (like any other data) are cultural products, socially produced by individuals or organisations with particular

priorities and ways of seeing the world (Macdonald 2008). Documents are *things* (Prior 2004) that require careful appraisal. Until the 1960s official statistics (such as unemployment levels and rates of suicide) were seen as objective measures of social events, but critical perspectives urge us to scrutinise the processes through which documents and datasets are produced. Documents may have been manipulated for particular purposes (White 2003). Corporations spend vast amounts of money trying to ensure their image and words are presented in particular ways, and therefore documents or data sourced from them must be examined carefully (May 2001). Therefore, researchers must be critical, reflect, and check against other sources for validity (McCulloch 2004).

2 *Date and timeliness.* Secondary data are never static: they are always being generated and (re)produced. Conversely, some datasets are cancelled and others are destroyed or deleted (Clark 2005). Furthermore, researchers need to ensure that documents or datasets are timely and relevant. For example, if the data are aged, do they (and how do they) have use and currency for your research?

3 *Purpose.* Secondary data have already been collected with original goals that may or may not mirror your own research aims. The original data collection process may have asked questions differently to your preferred phrasing (White 2003). Furthermore, the original data may not be available for analysis at the scale (local, regional, national or international) in which you are interested.

4 *Accessibility.* Whilst a huge range of sources of secondary research are available publicly, others may be held privately and so could be difficult or impossible to access. Many corporation reports may be available only internally, within organisations. Personal letters or memoirs may also be held in private collections and so not publicly available (Macdonald 2008). Other sources may be accessible only with special permission, which may require lengthy negotiation or trips to specific locations to access the data, have special conditions applied (e.g. no photocopying) or be pay-per-view. All of these conditions may thwart youth practitioners who have limited time and resources. Furthermore, reorganisation can result in records being lost, misplaced or misfiled, and organisations may find that specific records are inaccessible only once they have been asked for them. Storage formats also change at a rapid pace. For example, documents from the 1990s may be stored on floppy disks, which few PCs are now able to read (Clark 2005).

5 *Quality.* We often do not know the quality or robustness of secondary data. Critical methodological investigation is required, considering the choice and design of method (see Chapter 2), sampling approach, frame and sample size and the form of data processing, coding and initial analysis (see Chapter 6). Furthermore, errors made in the generation of data may be unknown to us. Attempts to evaluate the quality of data can be hampered by the lack of data production information, although increasingly government datasets contain this supplementary yet essential evidence.

6 *Authenticity.* Although we may be confident that government-generated data is authentic, in other cases (particularly historical or personal documents) we may wish to check authenticity. Whilst it is rare for people to forge entire documents (e.g. the 'Hitler Diaries'), mistakes and misattribution do happen. Key questions to

consider are whether sources are genuine, reliable and attributed to the right person? If there is more than one copy of the document, are they similar? How might you be able to account for any differences? Is your copy complete or are pages missing?

7    *Credibility*. This involves considering the integrity of the source and faithfulness of the account. Although complete fakery is rare, a source can be censored, biased or focused in particular ways (McCulloch 2004). Is the document free from distortions or error? Has a long time passed between the event and recording (Macdonald 2008)?

8    *Representativeness*. When evaluating sources, we need to consider both *selective deposit* (how representative the sources are of the event under investigation) and *selective survival* (which data/documents have been withheld for reasons of confidentiality, commercial sensitivity and so on). Consider the existence of other possible sources, which may complement or contrast with the chosen source. If only a few sources survive (and survival can be dictated by chance and haphazard), how much faith can we put in them?

9    *Meaning*. The meaning of secondary data can be assessed in a variety of ways. In a literal sense, familiarity with language of the author, intended audience, group or culture is needed. Various analyses offer a deeper consideration of meaning. It can be helpful to consider the text itself, the subtext (including the meanings drawn by a particular audience) and the context of its production.

## Analysing secondary data

There is no consensus about how 'best' to analyse secondary data (May 2001; Silverman 2006). Reflecting earlier discussions, different approaches to analysing data represent alternative ways of thinking about how to make sense of the world (McCulloch 2004). One approach is that secondary research forms the evidence through which we find out 'the truth' about an event. Two main forms of this type of analysis are used, depending upon the kind of data.

### Quantitative secondary data analysis

Quantitative secondary data analysis is broadly similar to analysis of primary quantitative data (see Chapter 6), although the former raises additional queries. We need to gather contextual information about the original collection of data, including how concepts were defined and operationalised: for example, how the dataset defined 'young person', 'school leaver' or 'service user'. Information about other methodological issues is needed, relating to sample size, response rate and data entry, cleaning, coding and processing (e.g. how the data were entered into a spreadsheet or database, how the responses were coded, whether any of the data were recoded, how the data were 'cleaned', and how any missing data – questions with ineligible responses or no response – were dealt with). All this information is needed to make judgements about the quality, validity and power of the findings generated from our secondary analysis. Some archives (for example, the ESDS and the Office for National Statistics) provide this contextual information, but be wary of large-scale datasets where it is not provided.

## Content analysis

Content analysis is one way to analyse the content of documents (and the more qualitative data within datasets: for example, open-ended questions). It seeks to identify patterns in the text objectively and often quantitatively (Kitchin and Tate 2000), and involves the systematic creation of a set of categories (a coding frame), followed by an analysis of the document to count the number of instances (e.g. words or phrases) that fall into those categories (Leveille and Chamberland 2010). However, the frequency of appearance of a category does not necessarily indicate its importance, so a more qualitative version of content analysis has been developed that explores the significance of categories through the use of illustrative examples. For example, Klingman and Shalev's (2001) content analysis of young people's graffiti uses a quantitative approach to count the number of references to particular discussions/events whilst also quoting in full some interesting but less typical examples of social commentary from young people to highlight the full spectrum of opinion.

However, content analysis has its critics. Predetermined categories are restrictive, as codes are constructed by researchers, rather than authors or audiences. Uncategorised events or activities are not recorded (Silverman 2006) and information that cannot be quantitatively measured and standardised is omitted (May 2001). Focusing on content can also reproduce the author's meaning, terms of reference and context, rather than looking critically at what has been said (or, perhaps more importantly, what has *not* been said).

## Towards a more critical approach to secondary data analysis

Increasingly, researchers have questioned whether documents or datasets offer the truth about events. Secondary data cannot be seen as facts, since they are not transparent records reflecting an external reality but *things* that are produced, manipulated and consumed (Prior 2004). Hence, secondary data becomes the topic under consideration, focusing on its style, form, the social context of its production and its purpose (McCulloch 2004). Macdonald's (2008: 286–287) discussion of documents can also be applied to other forms of secondary data, such as datasets:

> A document, like an untrustworthy witness, must be cross-examined and its motives assessed. How was it written, what was it really, why did it take place in that way, what was the point? Who had a motive? Who benefited? Who was in a position to write and disseminate it? Who was it intended to deceive and why?

This is not to say that secondary data aims to mislead or falsify deliberately, rather to acknowledge that it might not be objective (Macdonald 2008). To consider how documents and datasets are constructed involves looking at the production of intended meanings: what messages the data may intend to communicate and the arguments used to convince audiences. As May (2001: 195) comments, we can explore the processes by which 'documents try to stamp their authority upon the social world they describe'. Also, as readers do not simply accept the messages relayed to them, we need to be mindful of how documents are consumed and interpreted by audiences (Miller and Alvarado 2005). For example, reports or official statistics often have different impacts from those their authors or commissioners intend (McCulloch 2004). Therefore, secondary data are part of the way in which particular versions of truth and reality are produced (Wilson 2009). As Silverman (2006: 157) states: 'the role of textual researchers is not to criticize or to assess particular texts in terms of apparent "objective" standards. It is rather to analyse how they work to achieve particular effects.'

## Discourse analysis

One method of analysing text-based documents is *discourse analysis*. Although there are different kinds, these approaches all focus on the significance and structuring effects of language, and they are generally interpretive, reflexive styles of analysis (Burman and Parker 1993). A definition of a discourse is a set of terms and phrases that defines an object (Foucault 1972; Parker 1990). Discourse analysis attends to the need to consider the context for a document's production and use. Theoretical approaches informed by a Foucauldian understanding are usually concerned with the social and political implications of a text. They treat words as *not only* words by recognising their potential to construct or represent the world, and our choices within it, in particular ways. As youth practitioners, we are concerned with power and how people of different ages are positioned in relation to, say, entitlement to vote and understandings of 'maturity' or 'recklessness'. Burman and Parker (1993: 1–2) illustrate what a concern with power means in practice:

> Language organized into discourses . . . has an immense power to shape the way that people . . . experience and behave in the world. Language contains the most basic categories that we use to understand ourselves; affecting the way we act . . . When we talk about any phenomenon (our personality, attitudes, emotions), we draw on shared meanings (so we know that the listener will know what we are saying) . . . and contrasting ways of speaking [can be called] repertoires (Potter and Wetherell 1987) or discourses (Parker 1992) or ideological dilemmas (Billig *et al.* 1988).

A discourse analysis might help identify the political implications of a particular set of terms as they become popular in practice settings or identify the model of child development on which they rest. It is what a discourse does or how it functions that is of interest (Billig *et al.* 1988). Thus, what is said or written (or pictorially represented) is examined in terms of the social or political features of the discourse rather than simply the author/speaker's attitude or understanding. It is because these discourses 'do' things in the world (have concrete consequences for people's lives) that they are of interest. So the research question posed might be 'What is the significance of writing about young people in that way?' or 'What political views does/did this document sustain, promote or occlude?' For instance, what discourse of 'youth' is mobilised by flyers for events that misspell words or adopt graffiti-style fonts? Does this discourse construct a masculine, urban, 'cool' youth?

Whilst Parker's (1992) twenty-two steps for conducting discourse analysis are recommended, Alldred and Burman (2005) have simplified his approach to twelve stages, and Willig (1999) offers a three-step version:

1　Identify constructions being 'talked into existence'.
2　Identify 'subject positions' arising from these constructions.
3　Recognise how these constructions relate to other discourses.

As this indicates, a minimalist method of discourse analysis will involve: first, identifying constructions; second, identifying the ways individuals can be positioned within these understandings; and third, analysing how these understandings relate to discourse more widely.

In one collection of discourse analysis (Parker and the Bolton Discourse Network 1999), there are analyses of existing texts, such as children's literature, comic strips and advertisements, and of physical objects of study that need to be rendered textual before analysis (e.g. cities, gardens, playgrounds), as well as individual or group interview transcripts.

---

### Case study 7.2

### An example of discourse analysis

---

Alldred and David's (2007) discourse analysis of the policy document *Sex and Relationship Education Guidance* (DfEE 2000) is summarised here in relation to Willig's (1999) three steps.

## What constructions are talked into existence?

- *Sex and relationship education* (SRE) is constructed as an important area of learning that children 'need [in order to] live confident, healthy and independent lives' (p. 3), that must be taught in school 'in a moral framework' (p. 3) and that relates to 'difficult moral and social questions' (p. 3), implying that other areas of the curriculum do not raise such questions.
- *Sex* is constructed as negative and risky. It is presumed to be heterosexual and penetrative since the primary risk is pregnancy. Sex and relationship education should teach the 'reasons for delaying sexual activity' (p. 4).

- *Unplanned pregnancy* is constructed as unwanted, undesirable and pre-
  ventable by good education and appropriate decision-making. The only
  discourse of pregnancy is as 'unplanned and undesirable'.

It can be helpful to consider what is not said and alternative constructions. Sex
is not constructed as a potential enhancer of relationships or well-being. The
discourse of sex education is not one of human rights and entitlement, of the
right to either information or sexual autonomy, but one of risk reduction.

Another way to draw discourses into focus is historical comparison:
compared with thirty years ago, the issue of morality is foregrounded explicitly
(in pupils' moral choices) but, significantly, delivering sex and relationship
education within schools is constructed as the moral thing to do in order that
young people are 'supported', 'prepared' and 'protected'.

## What subject positions arise from the above?
## (Who is constructed?)

- *Young people* are understood as having certain needs, facing future
  decisions, on which they must deploy 'values', 'individual conscience' and
  'moral considerations' in order that their decisions are 'responsible and well
  informed' (p. 3). Their sexual desire is coyly referred to only as 'feeling
  attraction' (p. 25), and their sexuality is constructed as safely arising only
  in the future.
- *Pupils* are constructed as in need of protection from inappropriate teaching
  materials and their 'age and cultural background' are to be taken into
  consideration in teaching SRE. Technically the same constituency as 'young
  people' above, reference to 'pupils' is associated with discussions of puberty,
  maturation, developmentally appropriate materials and protection, and not
  with discussion of sexual desire or practice.
- *Parents* are constructed as people to be consulted (within a discourse of the
  values of 'parents, governors and the wider community'; p. 3), whose views
  schools should respect and whose values teaching should reflect. While
  parents' values are given status, pupils' 'views' (never 'values') are seldom
  mentioned and are to be attended to in order to promote self-esteem rather
  than because of their right to be heard or to influence provision.
- *Teachers* are referred to less frequently than parents (as demonstrated in a
  simple content analysis count).

Pupils are constructed as having been problematically gender differentiated in
the past: 'Traditionally the focus has been on girls. Boys may have felt that sex
education is not relevant to them and are unable or too embarrassed to ask
questions about relationships or sex' (p. 11). Pupils' needs are differentiated in
paragraphs about gender (above), ethnicity, special educational needs and
sexual orientation. Homosexuality, a contentious UK educational issue since

1988's Section 28, is framed only as a topic for discussion so that the needs of all pupils are met, rather than placing it legitimately on the curriculum for all.

## How do these constructions relate to other discourses?

An important aspect of discourse analysis is to 'go beyond the text' or to place discourses within wider politics. The handling of homosexuality reflects an individualist rather than a social justice approach – education is being tailored to meet individual needs, not to make society more just.

The negativity about sex and teenage pregnancy reflects the concerns of the Teenage Pregnancy Strategy (SEU 1999) that drew the renewed attention to SRE that produced this policy. Reflecting on the context of the document's production enables this link to be made, and following Parker's (1992) suggestion to consider the institutional consequences of a discourse highlights how sex education reflects and serves neoliberal concerns with the individual, with the financial consequences of individual behaviour, and with the management of risk.

For Parker (1992), the politics of language are important, and the final stages of his approach are concerned with tracing the political consequences of using a particular discourse: for instance, which social practices and institutions are supported. Ask whose interests are served by the use of that, as opposed to an alternative, discourse. The Alldred and Burman (2005) summary retains this emphasis, and, along with Harper's (2006) and Willig's (1999), is one of the shorter (chapter-length) descriptions of how to conduct discourse analysis. Combined with Case study 7.2 and Practice-based task 7.3, this offers a model of how to present discourse analysis.

## Practice-based task 7.3  Discourse analysis of a group discussion

Deborah Marks (1993) analysed a group discussion of an education case conference. The case conference is about 'Mike', a young black man, aged fourteen. His parents, teachers and other (white) welfare professionals discuss his exclusion in response to his 'behaviour problems' due to perceived 'problems at home'. Discourse analysis of the actual case conference challenged the way professionals defined the issues, but failed to leave space for Mike and his parents to contribute. Marks concluded that in place of idealised inter-professional communication, different interest groups employed rhetorical devices to promote specific interests.

Two years later, Marks undertook a group discussion with the same participants with the aim of supporting Mike and his family by showing how dominant discourses limited their participation by the way they were positioned in relation to powerful expertise. She also wanted to show how attitudes do not remain fixed in the individual and how conceptualising attitudes as discourses helps challenge people's ideas and beliefs.

From the transcript of the second discussion, Marks identified a set of references by various speakers to the benefits of taking part in the conference, of offloading, 'having your say', and of what is of support or help (emotionally) to Mike. Marks calls this the *therapeutic* discourse and problematises the way it functions to let the professionals parallel their own needs with Mike's, which serves to erase power differences. In addition, Marks identifies a *reflective* discourse that recognises different versions of events, such as the participants' varying interpretations and recollections of the previous meeting or their alternative understandings of racism. These two discourses can be in tension with each other and present different aims for the discussion.

1   Go to http://www.discourseunit.com/publications_pages/publications_books_dar.htm and download Marks's chapter (Chapter 8). Examine some of the extracts quoted. Can you see how different quotations, using different terms and phrases, and from differing participants, draw on the same discourse?

2   Are you convinced by Marks's description of the two discourses and of the text that she views as employing each?

3   Note how Marks demonstrates a discourse to the reader by the selection of multiple short extracts from the transcript. How many extracts are needed before you are convinced?

4   What is it possible to 'do'/argue with this type of analysis (and what is it not)?

## Ethics and secondary research

Most discussions of ethical principles focus upon primary data collection involving human participants. There has been far less discussion about the ethical use of documents and secondary data. Most higher education institutions do not require ethical approval for research solely comprising secondary research. However, that does not mean there are no ethical issues arising from conducting secondary research. Indeed, the same ethical principles apply (see Chapter 3). As secondary sources may include data that may have been collected by someone else or data not specifically generated for research purposes (e.g. discussions in an internet forum), we may want to be reassured that we are re-analysing data that have been collected ethically and that participants have consented to others viewing and analysing their responses. Current ethical guidelines suggest that researchers collecting primary data should communicate whether the data will be archived, the terms and conditions under which they will be shared, and gain consent (ideally in writing) for this from participants. However, if this assurance is not specifically stated in archives, it is difficult for secondary data users to know if it has been obtained. Also, completing ethical forms to the appropriate standard does not ensure that research was conducted in an ethical manner.

Furthermore, historical sources may well have been produced in a time and context where a concern for ethical practice was less of a priority. For example, whilst it is now convention that informed consent should be sought from young participants, research may not have sought this historically from young people. This raises ethical issues about using secondary data that we cannot be assured were obtained according to current ethical standards.

Guidelines also suggest that users of secondary data have the same ethical and legal obligations as primary data users, and even though the data may be in the public domain, researchers should assure anonymity and not disclose confidential or identifiable information. Practically, this may require us to consider how we might anonymise sources, including people, organisations and places. One dilemma is how we maintain anonymity whilst at the same time acknowledging individuals and institutions that have helped us by searching for or providing the data.

## Case study 7.3

### Ethics and secondary research

Francesca Moore's paper (Moore 2010) reminds us that secondary research (in common with all forms of research) can focus on sensitive topics. Moore's work researching women involved in abortion crimes in the late nineteenth and early twentieth centuries reminds us that even though data are already in the public domain, we are still required to act ethically in our use of such material. Using secondary data to study social practices that these women had desperately tried to keep hidden presents acute ethical dilemmas. As Moore discusses, it is impossible to know whether individuals would have consented to research being carried out on their behaviour nearly a hundred years later. Similarly, in contemporary research, although participants may have consented to transcripts of interviews being placed in an archive, it is debatable whether they were able to make a fully informed decision about data reuse, since participants can never fully know the nature or focus of future research projects.

Furthermore, Moore reminds us to be mindful that the public (re)release of information may cause distress to individuals, descendants of historical figures, or even (by association) broader communities or groups. She suggests that ethical practice in secondary research may include ensuring privacy and anonymity, for instance by changing the names of historical individuals (as even though they may be long dead, they can still be important figures in the local community) or places.

## Questions to consider

1  Do you think it is ethical for researchers to undertake secondary research that might 'uncover' that your direct ancestors or ancestors of members of your hometown participated in abortion crimes? How would you feel?

2  If we cannot secure informed consent from participants (because they are no longer alive, or because they are not traceable as we have only their anonymous transcripts downloaded from an archive), is it ethical to use their data for our own research purposes?

3  Should we anonymise individuals, organisations and places in historical research?

4  How can we undertake secondary research in an ethical manner?

## Summary of main points

- Secondary research is a very useful if not often considered way of conducting research. It offers youth practitioners access to data without requiring investment of time (by researcher or participants) in data collection stages.
- Secondary research takes many forms. Documents (including government reports, official records and organisational paperwork) are common sources. Large-scale datasets are another. Some may be quantitative (large-scale datasets), whilst others may be qualitative (often text based). Decisions about which form of secondary research to use are not just practical. They reflect broader debates about how to construct knowledge about the world.
- There is a huge variety of sources for secondary research. These include government agencies, local authorities, youth organisations and services, voluntary organisations and charities, community groups and individuals.
- There is growing awareness that documents and datasets are not objective measures of social events: they are socially produced. Secondary researchers need to treat them critically, as they are produced by particular individuals or groups and reflect their agendas as priorities. They are also exercises of power.
- There are different approaches to analysing secondary research. Some focus on exploring the content of sources, whilst others focus on the processes of production and intended meaning.

# Further reading

## *Documents*

Macdonald, K. (2008) 'Using documents', in N. Gilbert (ed.), *Researching Social Life* (3rd edn), London: Sage: 285–303.

McCulloch, G. (2004) *Documentary Research in Education, History and the Social Sciences*, London: Routledge Falmer.

Prior, L. (2004) 'Doing things with documents', in D. Silverman (ed.), *Qualitative Research Theory, Method and Practice*, London: Sage: 76–94.

## *Secondary data*

Allum, N. and Arber, S. (2008) 'Secondary analysis of survey data', in N. Gilbert (ed.), *Researching Social Life* (3rd edn), London: Sage: 372–393.

Clark, G. (2005) 'Secondary data', in R. Flowerdew and D. Martin (eds), *Methods in Human Geography: A Guide for Students Doing a Research Project*, Harlow: Pearson Prentice-Hall: 57–73.

May, T. (2001) *Social Research* (3rd edn), Buckingham: Open University Press.

## *Discourse analysis*

Alldred, P. and Burman, E. (2005) 'Analysing children's accounts using discursive analysis', in S. Green and D. Hogan (eds), *Researching Children's Experience: Approaches and Methods*, London: Sage: 175–198.

Parker, I. (1992) *Discourse Dynamics: Critical Analysis for Social and Individual Psychology*, London: Routledge.

Parker, I. (1994) 'Discourse analysis', in B. Banister, E. Burman, I. Parker, M. Taylor and C. Tindall (eds), *Qualitative Methods in Psychology: A Research Guide*, Buckingham: Open University Press: 92–107.

Parker, I. and the Bolton Discourse Network (1999) *Critical Textwork*, Buckingham: Open University Press.

Potter, J. and Wetherell, M. (1987) *Discourse and Social Psychology: Beyond Attitudes and Behaviour*, London: Sage.

# References

Alldred, P. and Burman, E. (2005) 'Analysing children's accounts using discursive analysis', in S. Green and D. Hogan (eds), *Researching Children's Experience: Approaches and Methods*, London: Sage: 175–198.

Alldred, P. and David, M. (2007) *Get Real about Sex: The Politics and Practice of Sex Education*, Buckingham: Open University Press.

Allum, N. and Arber, S. (2008) 'Secondary analysis of survey data', in N. Gilbert (ed.), *Researching Social Life* (3rd edn), London: Sage: 372–393.

Ansell, N., Barker, J. and Smith, F. (2007) 'UNICEF Child Poverty in Perspective Report: a view from the UK', *Children's Geographies*, 5 (3): 325–330.

Appleton, J. and Cowley, S. (1997) 'Analysing clinical practice guidelines: a method of documentary analysis', *Journal of Advanced Nursing*, 25: 1008–1017.

Atkinson, P. and Coffey, A. (2004) 'Analysing documentary realities', in D. Silverman (ed.), *Qualitative Research: Theory, Method and Practice*, London: Sage: 56–75.

Billig, M., Condor, S., Edward, D., Gane, M., Middleton, D. and Radley, A. (1988) *Ideological Dilemmas: A Social Psychology of Everyday Thinking*, London: Sage.

Burman, E. and Parker, I. (1993) 'Introduction: discourse analysis: the turn to the text', in E. Burman and I. Parker (eds), *Discourse Analytic Research*, London: Routledge: 1–13. Available at http://www.discourseunit.com/publications_pages/publications_books_dar. htm.

Clark, G. (2005) 'Secondary data', in R. Flowerdew and D. Martin (eds), *Methods in Human Geography: A Guide for Students Doing a Research Project*, Harlow: Pearson Prentice-Hall: 57–73.

DCSF (2003) *Every Child Matters*, London: HMSO.

DCSF (2005) *Youth Matters*, London: HMSO.

DFEE (2000) *Sex and Relationship Education Guidance*, London: HMSO.

Foucault, M. (1972) *The Archaeology of Knowledge*, London: Tavistock.

Gagen, E. (2000) 'Playing the part: performing gender in America's playgrounds', in S. Holloway and G. Valentine (eds), *Children's Geographies: Playing, Living, Learning*, London: Routledge: 213–229.

Gagen, E. (2004) 'Making America flesh: physicality and nationhood in early twentieth century physical education reform', *Cultural Geographies*, 11: 417–442.

Gagen, E. (2006) 'Measuring the soul: psychological technologies and the production of physical health in Progressive Era America', *Environment and Planning D: Society and Space*, 24: 827–849.

Harper, D. (2006) 'Discourse analysis', in M. Slade and S. Priebe (eds), *Choosing Methods in Mental Health Research*, London: Routledge: 47–67.

Kitchin, R. and Tate, J. (2000) *Conducting Research in Human Geography: Theory, Methodology and Practice*, Harlow: Prentice-Hall.

Klingman, A. and Shalev, R. (2001) 'Graffiti: voices of Israel youth following the assassination of the Prime Minister', *Youth and Society*, 32: 403–422.

Leveille, S. and Chamberland, C. (2010) 'Toward a general model for child welfare and protection services: a meta-evaluation of international experiences regarding the adoption of the Framework for the Assessment of Children in Need and Their families (FACNF)', *Children and Youth Services Review*, 32: 929–944.

Macdonald, K. (2008) 'Using documents', in N. Gilbert (ed.), *Researching Social Life* (3rd edn), London: Sage: 285–303.

Marks, D. (1993) 'Case-conference analysis and action research', in E. Burman and I. Parker (eds), *Discourse Analytic Research*, London: Routledge: 135–154. Available at http://www.discourseunit.com/publications_pages/publications_books_dar.htm.

May, T. (2001) *Social Research* (3rd edn), Buckingham: Open University Press.

McCulloch, G. (2004) *Documentary Research in Education, History and the Social Sciences*, London: Routledge Falmer.

Miller, F. and Alvarado, K. (2005) 'Incorporating documents into qualitative nursing research', *Clinical Scholarship*, 37 (4): 348–353.

Moore, F. (2010) 'Tales from the archive: methodological and ethical issues in historical geography research', *Area*, 42 (3): 262–270.

Papasolomontos, C. and Christie, T. (1998) 'Using national surveys: a review of secondary analyses with special reference to education', *Educational Research*, 40 (3): 295–310.

Parker, I. (1990) 'Discourse: definitions and contradictions', *Philosophical Psychology*, 3 (2): 189–204.

Parker, I. (1992) *Discourse Dynamics: Critical Analysis for Social and Individual Psychology*, London: Routledge.

Parker, I. and the Bolton Discourse Network (1999) *Critical Textwork*, Buckingham: Open University Press.

Potter, J. and Wetherell, M. (1987*) Discourse and Social Psychology: Beyond Attitudes and Behaviour*, London: Sage.

Prior, L. (2004) 'Doing things with documents', in D. Silverman (ed.), *Qualitative Research: Theory, Method and Practice*, London: Sage: 76–94.

Silverman, D. (2006) *Interpreting Qualitative Data: Methods for Analysing Talk, Text and Interaction*, London: Sage.

Social Exclusion Unit (SEU) (1999) *Teenage Pregnancy*, London: HMSO.

White, P. (2003) 'Making use of secondary data,' in N. Clifford and G. Valentine (eds), *Key Methods in Geography*, London: Sage: 67–85.

Willig, C. (1999) 'Discourse analysis and sex education', in C. Willig (ed.), *Applied Discourse Analysis: Social and Psychological Interventions*, Buckingham: Open University Press: 110–124.

Wilson, E. (2009) *School-based Research*, London: Sage.

## Useful websites

Australian Bureau of Statistics: http://www.abs.gov.au/
Central Statistic Office Ireland: http://www.cso.ie/
Economic and Social Data Service: http://www.esds.ac.uk/
Eurostat Information Service: http://epp.eurostat.ec.europa.eu/
UK National Archives: http://www.nationalarchives.gov.uk/
UK National Statistics: http://www.statistics.gov.uk
UNICEF's Child Info: http://www.childinfo.org/
US Census Bureau: http://www.census.gov/

# 8 Virtual and online research with young people

Nic Crowe

## Overview

> Every night I look at Facebook or World of Warcraft and see thousands of young people all happily interacting. Then I go to my youth centre and we have about six kids in. It's a no-brainer really. The web is where the kids are.
>
> (Natalie, youth worker)

For many youth workers, Natalie's observation is no doubt familiar and perhaps unsurprising. One of the most interesting popular cultural forms to emerge in recent years has been the range of digital online social spaces: social networking sites (e.g. Facebook), forums, chat rooms, online gaming arenas (such as World of Warcraft) and virtual worlds (Second Life, Twinity). Young people have always been early adopters of technology (Raine and Horrigan 2005) and these digital spaces now represent just another facet of their everyday experience (Livingstone 2009). In 2004, *UK Kids Go Online* noted that 70 per cent of all nine–nineteen-year-olds had regular access to the internet and on average spent more time engaged in online activities in a week than they would on homework (Livingstone and Bober 2004). By 2009, this figure had risen to 79 per cent (ChildWise 2009).

Over this brief period, digital communication technology became somewhat 'domesticated' and there is something very ordinary about the way in which many young people use it now. Technological space is one of a range of arenas they utilise, and young people are extraordinarily adept at moving between virtual and non-virtual (material) domains. The social networks facilitated by these virtual arenas have emerged as a central aspect of teenage life, forming part of a wider, more complex system of social interaction (Holloway and Valentine 2001). Conversations begun in the playground continue via phone and then move to chat rooms, MSM or Facebook. Digital technology offers new possibilities to transcend the confines of locality. New social networks have been formed, defined not by geography but rather by common interests or 'affinities' (Gee 2007), which bring together young people who would perhaps never have the opportunity to meet in non-virtual spaces. For these 'digital natives' (Prensky 2001), technologically created space is not special; it is just another place to 'hang out', meet friends, chat, just 'be'.

But this 'domesticity' sits in contrast to how the virtual world is treated by some researchers and many youth work and education practitioners. In much research there appears to be a trend to celebrate, indeed venerate, computer-mediated space as a socially disconnected field of study. New areas of research, for example into cyber-bullying, have often failed to see these as digital expressions of phenomena already present in the material world. Such manifestations should not automatically be treated discretely or separated from their material counterparts simply because the arena in which they are set is itself new. This is not to say that they should not be studied in their own right or that they do not have special characteristics, but it is easy to become side-tracked by the newness of the *spaces* themselves rather than concentrating on what is happening within them.

Conversely, risk-averse youth practitioners are often guilty of neglecting such spaces all together. With a few exceptions (Gee 2007; Squire 2005), education professionals have largely ignored the educational possibilities of digital spaces and too few youth services have chosen to engage young people online. There are, of course, exceptions: Swindon, Surrey and Wiltshire have all used virtual networks to enhance their work with young people, whilst the Youth Work Online project has provided an online resource for youth professionals interested in developing a digital dimension to their work. Perhaps some practitioners are scared off by popular anxieties about the technology rather than any professional understanding of the digital spaces themselves. Yet, as Natalie reminds us in the quote at the beginning of this chapter, this is precisely where we can find many young people, rather than in our centres and projects or on the streets. Digital spaces have begun to replace (or extend) some young people's traditional public arenas – the parks, malls and street corners – which have become increasingly risky and regulated places in which to hang out. Engaging with young people online is not intrinsically different from traditional notions of detached youth work. For those of us interested in understanding the everyday lives and experiences of young people, online space is an important area of study.

## Researching the digital natives

For many practitioner-researchers, undertaking a study in online space may be a daunting prospect. It might help from the outset if we can begin to see – in research terms, at least – online space as sharing many of the characteristics of material space. Elsewhere in this volume you have considered a range of methodological issues and methods of data collection. Digital expressions of these methods are equally applicable to virtual research fields: for example, virtual ethnography and participant observation, interviewing, content analysis and online surveys. Similarly, any virtual researcher will need to address methodological concerns, which are in essence similar to those that arise in non-virtual research. In this sense, the other chapters in this book are a useful and important starting point for research in virtual spaces. However, as is the case in all studies, individual research arenas throw up specific issues. In this chapter I want to explore some of these methodological and ethical issues that might be encountered by a new researcher engaged in qualitative research that considers how young people interact with these technologically created environments. In doing so I will focus on a six-year ethnographic study of an online virtual gaming world called Runescape to illustrate and clarify many of the issues identified.

## The 'language' of the virtual

Perhaps the major challenge for anyone engaging in online research is moving from meeting people 'in the flesh' of the material world to working in the 'insubstantiality' of the virtual (Mann and Stewart 2000). One of the main methodological issues in studying digital environments is that, unlike familiar modes of communication in the non-virtual world, participants communicating online have only text and very limited predetermined animations to convey personality, mood and emotions. Qualitative studies of virtual space, like those I discuss here, are concerned with social activity within a specific locality or context in which the virtual researcher must 'actively engage with people in online spaces in order to write the story of their situated context, informed by social interaction' (Crichton and Kinash 2003: 2). This research aims to help us understand the world in which we live and why things are the way they are. In short, it asks questions about the 'meanings' people bring to aspects of their everyday lives or situations. For those of us interested in understanding youth culture, this 'story' is expressed not only in terms of young people's lived experience but through the dimensions of 'agency' (the capacity of individuals to act independently and to make their own free choices) and 'identity' (how we consider aspects of 'self' in relation to our surroundings and others). These represent crucial aspects of young people's understanding of 'being in the world' and are central to any notion of *youth culture*, yet they can be properly understood only *relationally* as both *spatialised* and *placed* (Massey 2005: 184). Virtual space shares some characteristics with material space, having 'geography, physics, a nature and a rule of human law' (Benedikt 1991: 123) and, like material space, the virtual acts as a 'repository for cultural meaning – it is popular culture, its narratives created by its inhabitants that remind us who we are, it is life as lived and reproduced in pixels and virtual texts' (Fernback 1997: 37). Thus online spaces are not abstracted or isolated arenas. The virtual is not 'placeless' (Hillis 1999); rather, like all places, it is constituted by its own specific social practices.

So researching young people in the virtual world is, in one sense, not very different from studying them in the material world. All research arenas are simultaneously a physical location and a symbolic place. To see how this might be the case, let us think about the familiar location of a typical housing estate. If we wanted to research how young people made sense of living there, we would first consider aspects of the locality: we might study physical boundaries, amenities and popular meeting locations. But there would be other – perhaps less tangible – aspects of the estate that might also contribute to our understanding of what it means to live there: choice of language, dialect or slang used by particular groups; specific items of clothing that differentiate some residents of the estate from others; specific values or beliefs, or unique rituals/practices in which the young people are engaged. These form part of the 'symbolic' boundaries that define the estate and its meanings for people who live or hang out there. Such cultural 'markers' provide the substance of much qualitative research.

There is a potential challenge here for those of us engaged in online research. If we think about virtual space as being a digital manifestation of our typical estate, then many of these aural and visual cues – such as accents and clothing – that add depth to our virtual observations and interactions will be missing. Of course, this is more true of some digital spaces than others. Text-based environments, such as chat rooms, forums and peer2peer messaging, offer little beyond language to communicate any sense of meaning. Jones (1999) observes how in these instances a virtual researcher's field notes must provide details of the physical environment and both observations and impressions of how individuals and groups seem to experience, interpret and structure their lives. Such information adds additional depth and context to participants' words and actions. This, he argues, is not very different to the way in which qualitative researchers approach non-virtual research fields; even material researchers often have to rely on their participants' own language to describe or explain the context within which an action is taking place.

However, as Hall (1997) reminds us, such descriptions can never be completely value free since the environment or situation being described will itself have influenced the choice and style of the participants' language. This, in turn, can ascribe further meanings to the descriptions. So thinking again about our housing estate, dialects and accents may act as sub-cultural markers that allude to location, ethnicity or social class. The use of slang or jargon may point to affinity with a particular group or context. Any researcher should also note that language used may be sensitive to the researcher's own choice of language or the location within which the research takes place. For example, when I speak with young people in school settings, they often ask 'permission' to use certain words or apologise for swearing, something that is less common in less formal locations. Language is therefore used in different ways, for different purposes, in different situations.

New modes of discourse have emerged to help users 'fill in the blanks' and facilitate and structure social relations online. This 'language' of the virtual includes 'text speak' (e.g. 'cu l8er'), emoticons (e.g. '☺') and abbreviations (e.g. 'OMG', 'BRB', 'HMU', 'LOL'). Social networking sites offer slightly more sophisticated modes of discourse that might include photographs, video and certain forms of graphic interaction, all of which add depth to a researcher's consideration of participants. However, it is arguably the virtual worlds and online games that provide the richest and thickest data. These graphical environments offer the researcher an apparently more 'material' dimension than simple textual responses can give. As in material interactions, the researcher can observe 'in-world' (i.e. in the *game* world) behaviours and they are presented with a range of key cultural markers that carry capital *within* the world itself. These might include clothing, skill levels, class of character (for example a Wizard, Priest or Warrior in games that are based on medieval fighting and fantasy genres like World of Warcraft) and whether the participant owns or carries rare or high-status items. Furthermore, the representation of a participant's virtual body (or avatar) offers visible indications of choices of gender, race and so on.

Comparing this with day-to-day material settings, we can see how our race, gender and body size, occupation, social class, age, clothing, hairstyle, piercings or tattoos, even the car we drive combine to provide the raw material through which other individuals make judgements and assumptions of what we are like, what we do and where we come from. These markers help to provide the checks and balances needed to validate our assumptions and promote social life. Of course, sometimes these assumptions are incorrect or draw on prejudices and stereotypes, and they are usually based upon wider cultural values and assumptions.

Since virtual disembodiment separates the language of both researcher and participants from the material–social context that would give their words meaning, one of the frequent concerns from critics of virtual research is the question: how do you know to whom you are really talking? Virtual 'language' again plays an important interpretive role in this respect. But this is not really all that different from non-virtual research. Even in face-to-face material studies, researchers are often required to make subjective guesses. As Horn (1998: 91) observes, 'you don't have any more guarantees that someone is who they say they are just because you can see them. We are as often fooled by appearances as we are informed by them.'

Subjectivity is important in this respect and there is a rich history of seeing conceptions of the 'self' and 'other' in a fluid way. So, for example, what constitutes 'young' or what it might *mean* to be a 'young man' or a 'young woman' varies across cultures and from one historical moment to another. Individuals will tend to perceive the world in differing ways, so the same words spoken by each participant might not convey the same meaning. In virtual space the only information available about a participant is that which is generated by the digital world itself. Textual information or graphical representations provide all available data about the interaction as well as serving as the data themselves. Text must carry the social situation, but it must also carry the participants' relationships to the situation and their understandings of relationships between the knowledge and objects under discussion (Yates 1996: 46).

## Researching the virtual through the material

But there is also a need here to be careful in our interpretation of this virtual language. There is sometimes a tendency for new researchers to see the fluidity offered by digital space as a means to liberate participants totally from the fixity of material space. This is particularly true of virtual worlds that offer users the opportunity to experiment with alternative identities, roles and embodiments. Whilst it appears that the user can model their virtual bodies at will, they are in fact able to create a visual representation only from those that are available in the world. For example, in a virtual fantasy world such as World of Warcraft a young man can adopt the in-game persona of a 'young female wizard'. For some users, this form of identity experimentation will not move beyond a visual frame of reference, so to be a female character will be defined simply by conforming to dress codes – looking like a woman and dressing like a wizard. For others, there will be more sophisticated modes of play in which being 'a woman' is integral to a more extended form of role-play – for example, 'acting out' the part by adopting traditional female roles in the world. However, notions of gender here will be set by cultural dictates whether they are material – what it means to be a woman in the Western world in the early twenty-first century – or more developed popular cultural forms – what it means to be a woman in a fantasy environment. Either way, identity is not fixed internally but directed by external cultural norms and practices.

Virtual experience is at all times tethered in some fashion to material experience: 'The idea that you can isolate anything, any one piece of your life, and try to define it without referring to all that is connected to it is nonsense' (Horn 1998: 46). Whilst virtuality potentially removes the *control and consequential* elements of the material world, the cultural forces that help us make sense of material existence remain constant: we always come from somewhere. By logging into the virtual, an individual can represent himself/ herself as male or female, black or white, but their understanding of what it means to be a white man or a black woman will have been shaped by their cultural experience. Virtual spaces must therefore always be studied in relation to material space – or at least the everyday lived existence within which they are created and consumed.

## Case study 8.1

### Runescape

Up to now, I have been discussing methodological issues in a somewhat abstract manner. Perhaps the best way to appreciate the subtleties of virtual methods is to consider them in the context of a real study. For the past six years, I have been researching a small Java game-based world called Runescape, one of the new breed of 'free virtual worlds'. More commonly known as MMORPGs (massively multiplayer online role-playing games), the form is positioned midway between conventional online games and interactive visual chat, and is perhaps typified by the market leader, World of Warcraft. The emphasis is on role-play and character development rather than spatial progression, and there is considerable flexibility in the way that users can interact with the game narrative.

The worlds themselves are sophisticated multi-player interactions usually drawing on a familiar 'Tolkienesque' fantasy environment. World of Warcraft boasts 14.5 million accounts. In comparison, UK-based Runescape (1 million accounts and a regular UK base of 250,000 users) offers young people a less complex, although arguably no less challenging, virtual experience. Most interestingly, unlike its larger competitors, Runescape's user base consists almost exclusively of young people between the ages of twelve and eighteen – the demographic of most youth work projects.

When I began researching the space, I was interested in two main questions: first, I wanted to consider what uses young people are making of new online technological spaces, such as Runescape; second, perhaps more specifically,

I wished to investigate the extent to which Runescape offers young people a site where they can exercise both agency and communion. Whilst such questions may seem simple, they generate many sub-questions. What draws young people into, and sustains their interest in, these virtual arenas? Are such spaces merely 'entertainment space' or do they offer something more?

In order to address such questions and to understand the richness and complexities of Runescape, the most productive method of enquiry is to adopt an ethnographic-style participative observation approach (i.e. to 'play' the game). Hine (2005: 5) argues that this research method helps 'make explicit the taken for granted and often-tacit ways in which people make sense of their lives'. 'Playing the game' in any MMORPG also means accessing fan sites/forums and chatting to other players both online and in material spaces, such as meets and conventions.

## Virtual ethnography

Genzuk (2003) notes that an ethnographic approach is informed by three main methodological principles:

1   *Naturalism.* This stresses that research needs to take place in 'natural' settings – those that exist independently of the research process. This idea rejects the artificial nature of experiments or indeed arenas and settings set up principally as locations for research. It stresses first-hand contact with the phenomena under research as opposed to inferences from experiments or what participants say in interviews about what they do elsewhere. Naturalism also implies that social events, practices and processes can be explained in terms of their relationship to the context in which they occur. This implies that ethnographic researchers need to develop ways to reduce – or remove – the impact of their behaviour on the setting being studied. In this respect, participant observation is a particularly useful ethnographic method.
2   *Understanding.* This idea highlights a 'constructionist' perspective. Ethnography seeks to reject causal or mechanistic causality in terms of social behaviour, concentrating on the need to gain an understanding of the cultural perspectives on which behaviours are based.
3   *Discovery.* Ethnographic methods highlight a process of 'discovery' rather than one of 'testing' a specific idea or hypothesis. Thus, whilst research begins with a wider interest in certain social phenomena, it is subsequently focused as the research proceeds.

Hammersley (1990) identifies a range of 'key features' through which these themes are expressed:

•   People's behaviour is studied in everyday contexts, rather than under experimental conditions created by the researcher.

- Data are gathered from a range of sources, but mainly from observation and/or relatively informal conversations.
- The approach to data collection is 'unstructured' in the sense that it does not necessarily involve following through a detailed plan set up at the beginning; nor are the categories that are used for interpreting what people say and do predetermined or fixed. This does not mean that the research is unsystematic, simply that initially the data are collected in as raw a form, and on as wide a front, as is feasible.
- The focus is usually a single setting or group.
- The analysis of the data involves interpretation of the meanings and functions of human actions and mainly takes the form of verbal descriptions and explanations, with quantification and statistical analysis often playing a subordinate role.

As a set of methods, ethnography is not far removed from the sort of approach that we use in everyday life to make sense of our surroundings. Schwandt (1997: 60) notes, 'what constitutes data depends on one's enquiry purpose and the question one seeks to answer'. In the virtual world of Runescape, there is a wealth of data that helps us unpick how users make sense of their everyday virtual lives. In this sense, everything in Runescape constitutes data: choices of name; choices and 'looks' of avatars; choices of clothing and weapons/items carried; places that users choose to meet (or not meet); classes of characters and the special skills that users choose to concentrate on; social networks – both formal and informal – in which users engage; practices, rituals and institutions of the world. All these aspects of the virtual world help deconstruct its culture in a similar way to that of the material world.

One of the interesting aspects of virtual research across many arenas is that there appears to be a common and shared understanding of norms and common standards of online behaviours and language. Some writers (e.g. Rinaldi 1996) have argued that these form the ethical framework for online behaviour. 'Netiquette', as a concept, can be understood in two ways. First, it can mean a set of conventions and rules that structure all kinds of practice in online area – the norms and practices of the Runescape world, for example. Second, it is often used to refer to standards of courtesy in the virtual environment – such as not walking through another user's avatar. As a method of enquiry, participant observation helps maintain these expected modes of behaviour.

## Researching Runescape

In order to ensure the integrity of the Runescape virtual arena, it seems appropriate to use the main interactive tools of the world – its private and public 'chat' windows – as the main tools for data collection. The user interface displays in textual form all 'conversations' and interactions in the immediate vicinity. It also allows the user to talk privately with selected friends and contacts, all in textual form. The interactions are colour coded, which affords all parties some degree of tracking capacity, although this is very limited. (It would be worth you logging on to Runescape to see this.) The user interface keeps me in touch with my research arena in the sense that I can experience exactly what my co-participants are experiencing: I view events through the same 'window', hear the same sounds, see the same text. Like material ethnography, I 'live' in the world and, more crucially, I do not need to rely on second-hand interpretation since I am 'there'. The virtual ethnographer John Suler (1999) argues the strengths of such a subjective position. Whilst he acknowledges that this can reduce research objectivity, he notes that it is the very *subjectivity* of virtual ethnography that is its strength: 'one's thoughts and feelings . . . are refined into a powerful tool. By joining and participating in the group to be studied, the researcher becomes the very thing s/he is studying' (Suler 1999: 1). This reflexivity is, of course, fundamental to all good qualitative research.

One of the difficulties of attempting to access the world in this way is that the Runescape interface offers a very limited tool for complex interaction. On occasion, when more complicated or private responses are required, I use additional peer2peer technology: namely, Microsoft Messenger (MSM). This is mainly for practical reasons: during busy periods of interaction it is extremely hard to follow the thread of a conversation using the in-game communication (it is not designed for long and complicated interactions, such as interviews, and popular locations can get extremely busy with over a hundred separate conversations). MSM allows several conversation 'windows' to be open at once and it is possible to speak with several participants in a structured and organised way. Furthermore, it offers the facilities for 'group chat' where several people can share in and join a conversation. Interestingly, it is for this reason that some of the in-world communities, such as clans and guilds, use this method to coordinate their collective actions.

In this sense, the use of peer2peer could be considered a normalised Runescape activity for some types of user. However, I acknowledge that peer2peer also removes the subject from the field, and there is the criticism that my virtual interactions merely become disembodied text and subject to the concerns I outlined earlier. I think, in this case, the practical reasons for doing this outweigh the more philosophical criticism. The peer2peer interviews are used only for participants with whom I have a well-established virtual and often material relationship, and in cases where I feel comfortable about their virtual identity and character. This means that I can trust their interpretation of the events they are describing. I reason that it is a little like talking on the telephone with someone you know well.

My in-world interactions were all text based. I found that in Runescape's chat windows, as in those of other online games and worlds, text tended to follow the rules of conversation, rather than the formality usually associated with writing. Thus I considered typos and other mistakes to be more acceptable because I saw them as the textual equivalent of 'umming and ahhing'. Similarly, slang ('ROFL' – 'rolling on the floor laughing'), phonetic writing ('2day', 'B4') and the use of emoticoms (':P', '☹' ) were also acceptable, since they helped fill in some of the missing context I discussed earlier. When I present these kinds of data, wherever possible I quote text as it appeared rather than attempt to 'edit' or 'correct' it. Such an approach contrasts with the more formal exchanges that might be expected in email or forum posts, for example.

## Public or private?

However, my reliance on the main interface raises a key methodological issue: namely, whether what is 'said' online is 'public' or the 'property' of individual authors whose collection as 'data' requires consent in the first place (Hine 2000: 25). As in material space, virtuality is defined by the 'public' status of its interactions. Conversations in Runescape occur through text-based interaction that is 'the essential and most common element of virtual ethnography' (Crichton and Kinash 2003: 2). This is not very different from material ethnography. The young people interviewed in my research discussed how they used Runescape and other virtual spaces, such as MySpace, as arenas within which to define self through text, and, equally importantly, to seek *public responses* from peers through comments and messaging. In such arenas, messages and in-world texts form integral parts of the process of mutual identification.

Wright *et al.* (2002) observe that *public* interaction between users is a fundamental feature of all online games and worlds. Interaction in Runescape is a public activity. The interface window displays all conversations between users, and the openness – the 'public status' – of what is said is accepted and acknowledged by all users. Homan (1991) argues that whether a space is public or private is always relative to the definitions of those who occupy it, and this resonates with the idea of virtual communities, where there are no pre-existing cultural understandings of the nature of the media to appeal to or be guided by in defining the situation. But, as Goffman (1971) acknowledges, the 'private' always exists within a public arena. In Runescape, the two realms are clearly delineated by accepted practices. Whilst the main 'chat' interface is considered public – words appear in both the main game window above the characters who spoke them and in the conversation log directly below it – there is also a facility for 'private chat' which is visible only to those in the conversation loop. This appears as a different-coloured, superimposed text on the main game window.

This delineation between public and private aspects of play is well developed across all online worlds, particularly in games where there is some form of oppositional play against other teams or individuals. It is not too different from material-based systems used by the military or sports teams. In Runescape, the phrase 'move to private' is a well-established protocol and indicates that users no longer wish to be 'heard'. Conversely then, it is legitimate to infer, whatever is not limited to the private channels is intended for public consumption.

## Anonymity, consent and trusting your experience

It is clear that the vast majority of my data are obtained from in-game observations and discussions. These are enhanced in the virtual realm by more extended and developed discussions and interviews using other virtual arenas. Of these, nearly half are with separate individuals and mostly via casual in-game encounters. Runescape is a tight community with each server holding approximately 2,000 users; as many of the members stick to a particular server, it is easy to build up in-game relationships with other players simply because I encounter them daily.

I have to rely on trust and intuition in relation to participant age and gender. Many virtual worlds do not keep (or will not disclose) demographic details of their user base. There is often no mechanism to verify whether the details given to me by the young people are accurate or 'truthful'. Many writers have stressed that material identity is not fixed or given, thus similar constraints cannot be imposed within the virtual world. However, even though what it *means* to be a young man or young woman is arguably fluid, the sex and age of my participants are fixed by biological factors.

Since my research seeks to make claims about the online presence and activities of *young* people, I want to employ some devices to support the accuracy or robustness of this area of data.

Thompson (1988) observes that in conducting research we attempt to establish the truth in three ways: through reasoning, research and our personal experiences. Cohen *et al.* (2000) extend this idea, claiming that the three approaches are overlapping and complementary. Van Dalen (1973) suggests that when confronted with a problem we call upon our personal knowledge to help solve it through an appeal to our past experiences. I undertake my research with nearly twenty years of teaching and youth work experience of working with this age group, combined with considerable gaming and virtual social-networking proficiency. I believe that this gives me a sound base from which to judge whether the participants I am interacting with are really who they say they are. Of course, some 'adults' might well have slipped through the net, but this is also a feature of virtual space. The role-play aspect of these worlds allows some adults occasionally to represent themselves as young people. This is similar to the ways in which young people sometimes attempt to pass themselves off as adults in material space.[1] Such 'deceptions' might occur for a variety of reasons (not all of them sinister) and researchers should not be afraid to call upon their trust and experience to make judgement calls; indeed, as professionals working with young people, this is often one of our methodological and professional strengths.

Earlier, I discussed the difficulties associated with using data from public arenas and noted how in virtual spaces the 'public' nature of the interaction raises ethical and methodological issues. One such area centres on participant anonymity. I take the view that such 'public' consumption need not challenge participant anonymity or confidentiality. Most youth professionals will be familiar with the need for maintaining the confidentiality of young people, and the methods employed in virtual conversations would be similar to those used in more familiar youth work interactions. In research it would be usual in a study that quotes directly from young people to maintain their anonymity either by changing names or by using other mechanisms of disguise, such as 'Young Person A'. Although it could be argued that virtual names hide material identity, I feel that a user's on-screen name is an integral (and perhaps the most tangible) aspect of their virtual identity. Many of the participants in my study know that I am recording their responses and as with any research I seek their consent to use their words. Where I record more casual interactions it is impossible to obtain permission from participants in the usual way and I am forced to change their names to maintain their anonymity. As many users choose their names carefully as an extension of their online personas, I want to maintain a sense of this in my recordings of their words and actions. I have therefore begun to use names that still capture the essence of their identities. I accept that this is researcher intervention, but I justify it in terms of maintaining the tone and feel of the interaction and as an acknowledgement of the young person's unknowing contribution to my work.

Issues of *informed consent* are often less straightforward and in ethnographic studies this is a particularly problematic area. Some aspects of virtual research can borrow practices from material research. For participants in material interviews and focus groups, it is easy to obtain a standard hard-copy consent form signed by a parent or guardian where appropriate. This is sometimes less easy in online interactions and often the researcher is required to adopt a 'best-fit' or 'situated' approach. For example, when I contact participants via peer2peer technology, I always obtain an electronic copy of my permission form, again verified by a parent or guardian. Of course, I have to take this aspect on trust, but this is not intrinsically different to material 'signed' consent forms. Unless we see them being signed, or check with parents/guardians personally, do we have any way of knowing that the signatures are genuine?

In line with the points I made earlier in the chapter, I take the position that forum posts are in the public arena. If I want to use any of these data, I simply email the correspondent and ask permission to use their posting, usually via the forum itself, since only a few forums display personal email details. Where this is impossible, I try to use the data only in a more general way and ensure anonymity using the previously detailed methods.

## Ethical guidelines

In-world interactions fall into three groups:

1  Casual interactions and observations – what might be described as 'non-disclosed' participative observation – clearly cannot give informed consent but they are still valid within this sort of research. Such encounters are almost impossible to track down after they have taken place, but I attempt to let users know what I am doing by posting on the in-game forums – regular meeting places for most users. I again ensure anonymity, as detailed earlier.
2  Developed in-game encounters, such as long conversations or meetings over a short period of time. In such cases I might obtain consent via the in-game chat log, since securing email permission is not practical.
3  Sustained in-game interactions are treated in the same way as peer2peer participants (i.e. using an electronic consent form). I choose this method where I feel safety and/or ethical issues make this more appropriate than communication outside of the game or where the nature of the encounters makes other methods less practical. Given current anxieties about online grooming, this is particularly important to ensure the safety and integrity of both adult researcher and young participant(s).

I am sure that many youth practitioners will see parallels here with familiar ethical and professional guidelines for acceptable practice with young people. It is important that we stay mindful of these when attempting to research young people online. There is considerable guidance in terms of safeguarding children participating in material research and these provide an important starting point for virtual studies. The Association of Social Anthropologists (ASA) produces ethical guidelines for researching 'vulnerable groups' but these make no specific mention of children. The British Sociological Association suggests researchers seek expert help when dealing with young people and vulnerable groups. As yet, neither professional association has addressed researching children online directly. Interestingly, the National Children's Bureau (NCB) has recommendations that closely mirror those of the ASA and briefly touch on computer and online interactions, although it is more concerned with child protection than with the ethics of social research.

But perhaps we do not need to look to such institutions for guidance. As I noted earlier, as experienced youth practitioners, we are perhaps more aware of these issues and well used to what constitutes 'good practice' in terms of interactions with young people. Morrow (2005) observes that such guidelines are a little unhelpful in that they tend to raise questions about whether young people are competent to give 'informed consent' to the research process. This, she argues, is not a particularly empowering position to adopt towards young people. Mayall (1994: 11) adds an interesting dimension to the ethics debate when she observes that it is not the method of data collection that should come under scrutiny, but the subsequent analytical process and the use to which those data are put: while 'one might involve children in considering data, the presentation of it is likely to require analysis and interpretations for some purposes that . . . demand different knowledge than that generally available to children . . . in order to explicate children's social status and structural positioning'. Waksler (1991) suggests that this process undermines the status of young people in research since it locates adults as the sole articulators of the motives and structures behind the behaviour of young people; we should view young people as 'different' in their competencies, rather than less able.

## Power and status

Some interesting questions of power and status are raised here. It might be argued that there is a similar imbalance of power between researcher and participant within material research. Murphy and Dingwall (2001) note that the researcher occupies a powerful position since it is they who decide what is to be studied, how it should be researched and ultimately how it is written up and presented. This implies little participation and inclusivity in the research process. O'Reilly (2009: 60) argues that 'awareness of the potential for exploitation and the role of representation is the first step in trying to avoid it'. Certain forms of qualitative research, such as ethnography and other forms of participant observation, are not only particularly appropriate for studying virtual spaces but might offer less exploitative methods of enquiry in that they stress the need for relationships based on trust and rapport – again, something with which most youth practitioners will be familiar. Researchers using these methods often adopt a naturalist position. They listen to participants and attempt to understand their worlds through their own points of view. However, as Gledhill (1994) notes, it is important to recognise that, within this process, researchers still have control and influence over the data, and there have been instances when research has been accused of 'othering and exoticising its object' (O'Reilly 2009: 60).

Research based on Runescape raises interesting questions about the relationship between researcher and participants. In its virtual arena, power and status are not articulated in the same way as they are in the material world. Skill levels, class of character and possession of virtual goods form the social and cultural capital upon which status and reputation are based. There were many occasions, early in my research, when participants had far more developed characters than my own and thus occupied a more 'powerful' position within the Runescape world. As demonstrated by this example, many users were not afraid to exercise this power:

> I will answer your questions Nic, when you have made your bones. Come see me then and we can talk about it – ZamJam

ZamJam's assertion that he will speak to me only when I have 'made my bones' (proved my worth in the virtual world) illustrates that power is not always vested with the researcher. Indeed, the relationships of trust and rapport upon which participative methodologies are based are not afforded automatically; they have to be negotiated and won.

Interestingly, power, status and reputation, although based on virtual attributes, are actualised within both in-world and off-world practices. I found that in some cases this power framework extends beyond the confines of the virtual, as demonstrated by this extract from a material-based discussion:

> Helzbelle: But you wouldn't understand that Nic as you are just a 'noob'
> Nic: I am actually level 40 Helz
> Helzbelle: (laughs) Everyone under 60 is a noob to me, I worked hard to get there
> Justinjustout: Helz, you are the first 'legend' I have spoken to
> Helzbelle: Justin, you noob, shut it, you shouldn't even be speaking to me
> Basketbail: That's not fair Helz, everyone needs to get a chance to have their say
> Helzbelle: No, on Runey, he couldn't come up to me . . . I got a legends cape and its not 'allowed'
> Justinjustout: But we not on Rune you noob
> Helzbelle: What that got to do with it. You are still a noob whatever
> BonBon: She is right Nic, you just can't do that. You should apologise Justin
> Nic: Does everyone agree?
> (General agreement)

This exchange demonstrates how virtual power and influence become actualised in material-based research instances. Helzbelle's status as a 'Runescape legend' extends beyond the confines of the virtual world, and the other participants in the discussion are expected to defer to her authority as a high-end player in the same way as they would within the world itself. This power relationship overrides all other power structures that might have originated in the material world, such as age (Helzbelle was one of the youngest in the group) or my status as an 'adult' (I was her youth worker) or a 'researcher' (all the participants had been involved in previous focus groups). There was a general consensus on her authority. Helzbelle was a young person who had 'made her bones' and was to be respected as such.

But, as O'Reilly (2005) rightly points out, in most cases the power of *representation* ultimately lies with the researcher. Closely associated with this is a need to address the degree of anonymity afforded by virtual arenas to the researcher. There is a long history of covert or semi-covert methods in qualitative research, particularly those strands that involve participant observation, yet it appears to be rarely justified and at best tolerated. Covert data collection is often presented in an emotive way, implying something 'underhand' or deceitful. But as a 'practice' it covers a range of method-ological approaches – from deliberate misrepresentation of the researcher to operating outside of 'informed consent' – some of which seem in tension with these negative connotations of the term.

There are practical difficulties in declaring oneself within many virtual arenas, not least when the virtual is afforded a different research status from that of the material. Garton *et al.* (1999: 93) question whether researchers must 'identify themselves if they are only participating in the electronic equivalent of hanging out on street corners or doughnut shops where they would never think of wearing large signs identifying them-selves as "researchers"'. As with much writing about technologically created space, concern about 'virtual anonymity' has more to do with anxieties about the medium itself than with any substantive ethical complexities that might arise.

## Participant risk

Research in virtual space is no more likely to 'misuse' data or harm participants than its material counterpart. Even in studies based in the material world, explicit research practice does not necessarily mean that participants will be aware of data collection or the use to which those data is put. This places the emphasis on individual studies and researchers, which in itself is not conducive to the development of a wider set of prin-ciples. As more studies are undertaken, they will eventually contribute to the precedents and experience of virtual research. Yet even these precedents do not guarantee clarity. Material-based research does not always explicitly declare whether permission was obtained. Denzin (1999) admits that in some of his early virtual research he operated covertly and did not seek permission to use forum posts (indeed, from whom would he ask permission, especially given that some 'virtual identities' are transitory?). As Reid (1996) acknowledges, the lack of clear guidelines forces virtual researchers to make their own judgements on how best to interpret these precedents.

Adler *et al.* (1986: 367) note that covert research can be seen as deliberately deceptive because it is a role in which 'the researcher disguises the purpose and interest behind his or her participation at the scene'. But there is a significant qualitative difference between 'not declaring' and 'disguising'. It is the distinction between omission rather than commission: what I have done and what I have failed to do. Furthermore, within many online spaces, particularly virtual worlds and online games, the ideas of disguise and deception are perhaps not as clear cut as they might be in other spaces.

Since 'the non-disclosure of research identity in computer-mediated communication research appears to be an unresolved issue' (Sanders 2005: 71), can it be argued that participants are being placed in undue harm by undisclosed research? A quick glance at the ethical guidelines from many institutions seems to suggest that this might be the case. The fear of 'participant risk' is a key aspect in concerns about non-disclosure, particularly in an environment involving young people. I am not sure that the virtual environment itself provides any more risks than might be experienced in a material environment. Yet it might be that the participant's *perception* of what it means to be situated in the virtual could set up an ethical dilemma for the researcher. Coomber (1997) argues that the relationship between private and public online is ambiguous and, consequently, participants in virtual research could be 'tricked' into performing illegal activities. This is a pertinent observation and might certainly apply to social-networking arenas such as MySpace and Facebook where the private (or corporate) ownership of the technology is masked by a belief that it constitutes public space. In virtual worlds this is often less of a problem. 'In-world' controls, such as moderators and conversation filters, usually prevent offensive and illegal activity. Moreover, there is a tacit recognition that the creators of the world are always in the background to 'police' online activity. In many ways this is again similar to material society.

The Runescape research offers a good example of some of the methodological tensions present in studying virtual spaces. Sharf (1999) warns that the virtual provides a greater danger when dealing with sensitive or personal information since the technology does not afford the researcher the degree of control that they might have in the material. In relation to Runescape, I do not believe this to be the case, as I have demonstrated virtual research shares much in common with its material counterpart. Whilst I do not think that virtual participants endure any greater risks than they might in similar material research arenas, I think that Sharf's warning speaks to a particular attitude to the participant's relationship with the technology that brings our methodological argument full circle.

As researchers, we have become adept at operating within material spaces, but we are only just beginning to understand the implications of working within the virtual. Online arenas are accused of facilitating deceptions because many of the familiar cues that normally assign roles, and permit or inhibit participation, are not present. But, similarly, the material world offers opportunities for deceptions that would not be present in the virtual. So, the material – the embodied me – gives me the capacity to do some things that I could not do if I were not material. Unlike the material, where participants are largely known to each other, at least on a visual level, in the online environment such recognition does not necessarily occur. Users of virtual spaces can change the way they express their personalities, switch genders, change their age, or become fantasy characters in virtual worlds. As consistency in identity has strong associations with authenticity, these possibilities have clear implications for data. As a new arena for social research, the virtual will always be open to criticism and anxiety about its appropriateness as a research setting, its methods of data collection and the role and risks of its participants.

## Summary points

In this chapter I have considered the key ethical and methodological issues that might affect research into virtual spaces. Specifically, I looked at the following:

- Young people's use of virtual spaces. I observed how the virtual was becoming increasingly mundane and domestic as young people creatively reconfigured the space as an arena in which they extended what were formally material rituals and practices.
- The connections between the virtual and the material, and suggested that many of the methodological issues that arise in virtual research are not intrinsically different from those that we might encounter in material studies.
- Some strategies for researching in virtual arenas and outlined some of the ethical dilemmas that might face a researcher who is new to online spaces.
- A case study (Runescape) that I used to illustrate my earlier points and suggested might serve as a starting point for future research and interest.

### Practice-based task 8.1  Virtual and online research

Speak to a group of young people you know or work with.

- What sort of digital spaces do they use and what do they do when they are there? Why might these digital spaces be attractive?
- Can you help them make connections between their digital and material activities?

Log into a virtual world, such as Second Life (www.secondlife.com) or Runescape (www.Runescape.com).

- What do you consider the key methodological issues that might arise for researchers in this sort of world?
- Try to use the world regularly for two months and then revisit your initial assessment. Have your ideas and thoughts changed?

## Further reading

Boellstorff, T. (2008) *Coming of Age in Second life: An Anthropologist Explores the Virtually Human*, Princeton, NJ: Princeton University Press.
ChildWise (2009) *The Monitor Report 2008–9: Children's Media Use and Purchasing*, Norwich: ChildWise.

Crowe, N. and Bradford, S. (2006) 'Hanging out in Runescape', *Children's Geographies*, 4 (3): 331–346.

Gee, J.P. (2007) *Good Video Games and Good Learning: Collected Essays on Video Games, Learning, and Literacy*, New York: Peter Lang.

Hine C. (ed.) (2005) *Virtual Methods: Issues in Social Research on the Internet*, Oxford: Berg.

Jones, S. (1999*) Doing Internet Research: Critical Issues and Methods for Examining the Net*, Thousand Oaks, CA, and London: Sage.

Kendall, L. (1999) 'Recontexualizing cyberspace: methodological considerations for online research' in S. Jones (ed.), *Doing Internet Research*, Thousand Oaks, CA, and London: Sage, 57–75.

King, G. and Krzywinska, T. (2006) *Tomb Raiders and Space Invaders: Videogame Forms and Contexts*, London: I.B. Tauris.

Livingstone, S. (2009) *Children and the Internet: Great Expectations, Challenging Realities*, Cambridge: Polity Press.

Morrow, V. (2005) *Ethical Research with Children*, London: Open University Press.

Taylor, T.L. (2006) *Play between Worlds: Exploring Online Gaming Culture*, Cambridge, MA: MIT Press.

## Note

1   Many young participants in this study admitted to pretending to be older in order to buy alcohol. One had even claimed to be a parent in a telephone conversation with his school in order to get a friend the day off.

## References

Adler, P.A., Adler, P. and Rochford, E. (1986) 'The politics of participation in field research', *Urban Life*, 14: 363–376.

Benedikt, M. (1991) 'Cyberspace: some proposals', in M. Benedikt (ed.), *Cyberspace: First Steps*, Cambridge, MA: MIT Press, 119–224.

ChildWise (2009) *The Monitor Report 2008–9: Children's Media Use and Purchasing*, Norwich: ChildWise.

Cohen, L., Manion, L. and Morrison, K. (2000) *Research Methods in Education*, 5th edn, London: Routledge Falmer.

Coomber, R. (1997) 'Using the internet for survey research', *Sociological Research Online*. http://wwwsocresonline.org.uk/socresonline/2/2/2.html (downloaded 23/5/2004).

Crichton, S. and Kinash, S. (2003) 'Virtual ethnography: interactive interviewing online as method', *Canadian Journal of Learning and Technology*, 29 (2). http://www.cjlt.ca/content/vol29.2/cjlt29-2_art-5.html (downloaded 1/11/2010).

Denzin, N. (1999) 'Cybertalk and the method of instances', in S. Jones (ed.), *Doing Internet Research: Critical Issues and Methods for Examining the Net*, London: Sage, 107–125.

Fernback, J. (1997) 'The individual within the collective', in S. Jones (ed.), *Virtual Culture, Identity and Communication in Cybersociety*, London: Sage, 7–35.

Garton, L., Haythornthwaite, C. and Wellman, B. (1999) 'Studying online networks', in S. Jones (ed.), *Doing Internet Research*, London: Sage, 75–105.

Gee, J.P. (2007) *Good Video Games and Good Learning: Collected Essays on Video Games, Learning, and Literacy*, New York: Peter Lang.

Genzuk, M. (2003) *A Synthesis of Ethnographic Research*, Occasional Papers Series, Center for Multilingual, Multicultural Research, Rossier School of Education, University of Southern California. http://wwrcf.usc.edu/~genzuk/Ethnographic_Research.html (downloaded 3/8/2008).

Gledhill, J. (1994) *Power and its Disguises: Anthropological Perspectives on Politics*, London: Pluto Press.

Goffman, E. (1971) *Relations in Public: Microstudies of the Public Order*, Harmondsworth: Penguin.

Hall, S. (1997) *Representations: Cultural Representations and Signifying Practices*, London: Sage.

Hammersley, M. (1990) *Reading Ethnographic Research: A Critical Guide*, London: Longman.

Hillis, M. (1999) *Digital Sensations: Space, Identity and Embodiment in Virtual Reality*, Minneapolis: University of Minnesota Press.

Hine, C. (2000) *Virtual Ethnography*, London: Sage.

Hine, C. (ed.) (2005) *Virtual Methods: Issues in Social Research on the Internet*, Oxford: Berg.

Holloway, S.L. and Valentine, G. (2001) 'Placing cyberspace: processes of Americanization in British children's use of the internet', *Area*, 33: 153–160.

Homan, R. (1991) *The Ethics of Social Research*, Harlow: Longman.

Horn, S. (1998) *Cyberville: Clicks, Culture and the Creation of an Online Town*, New York: Warner Books.

Jones, S. (1999) *Doing Internet Research: Critical Issues and Methods for Examining the Net*, Thousand Oaks, CA, and London: Sage.

Livingstone, S. (2009) *Children and the Internet: Great Expectations, Challenging Realities*, Cambridge: Polity Press.

Livingstone, S. and Bober, M. (2005) *UK Children Go Online: Final Report of Key Project Findings*, London: Economic and Social Research Council.

Mann, C. and Stewart, F. (2000) *Internet Communication and Qualitative Research*, London: Sage.

Massey, D. (2005) *For Space*, London: Sage.

Mayall, B. (ed.) (1994) *Children's Childhoods: Observed and Experienced*, London: Falmer Press.

Morrow, V. (2005) *Ethical Research with Children*, London: Open University Press.

Murphy, E. and Dingwall, R. (2001) 'The ethics of ethnography', in P. Atkinson, A. Coffey, S. Delamont, J. Lofland and L. Lofland (eds), *Handbook of Ethnography*, London: Sage, 220–233.

O'Reilly, K. (2005) *Ethnographic Method*, London: Routledge.

O'Reilly, K. (2009) *Ethnography*, London: Sage.

Prensky, M. (2001) 'Digital natives, digital immigrants', *On the Horizon*, 9 (5). http://www.marcprensky.com/writing/Prensky%20-%20Digital%20Natives,%20Digital%20Immigrants%20-%20Part1.pdf (downloaded 3/7/2010).

Raine, L. and Horrigan, J. (2005) *A Decade of Adoption: How the Internet Has Woven Itself into American Family Life*, Washington, DC: PEW Internet and Family Life.

Reid, E. (1996) 'Informed consent in the study of online communities: a reflection on the effects of computer mediated social research', *The Information Society*, 12 (2): 169–174.

Rinaldi, A. (1996) 'The ten commandments for computer ethics', *The Net: User Guidelines and Netiquette*. http://www.fau.edu/netiquette/net/index.htm (downloaded 1/12/2007).

Sanders, T. (2005) 'Researching the online sex work community', in C. Hine (ed.), *Virtual Methods: Issues in Social Research on the Internet*, Oxford: Berg, 66–79.

Schwandt, T. (1997) *Qualitative Enquiry: A Dictionary of Terms*, London: Sage.

Sharf, B. (1999) 'Beyond netiquette: the ethics of doing naturalistic research on the internet', in S. Jones (ed.), *Doing Internet Research: Critical Issues and Methods for Examining the Net*, Thousand Oaks, CA: Sage, 243–256.

Squire, K. (2005) 'Changing the game: what happens when video games enter the classroom', *Innovate: Online Journal of Education*, August/September. http://www.innovateonline.info (downloaded 18/6/2010).

Suler, J. (1999) 'One of us: participant observation research at the palace', in J. Suler, *The Psychology of Cyberspace*. http://www.rider.edu/suler/psycyber/psycyber.html (downloaded 06/06/2006).

Thompson, P. (1988) *The Voice of the Past: Oral Histories*, Oxford: Oxford University Press.

Van Dalen, D. (1973) *Understanding Educational Research*, New York: McGraw-Hill.

Waksler, F. (1991) *Studying the Social World of Children: Sociological Readings*, London: Falmer Press.

Wright, T., Boria, E. and Breidenbach, P. (2002) 'Creative player actions in FPS online video games: playing counter-strike', *International Journal of Computer Game Research*, 2 (2). http://www.gamestudies.org/ (downloaded 4/4/2010).

Yates, S. (1996) 'Oral and linguistic aspects of computer conferencing', in S. Herring (ed.), *Computer-Mediated Communication: Linguistic, Social and Cross-Cultural Perspectives*, Amsterdam: John Benjamins, 24–46.

# Presenting research to different audiences

## Judith Bessant and Rys Farthing

## Overview

More than ever, good youth practice depends on being able to research 'issues' and then thoughtfully apply your 'discoveries'. Applied research is a core skill for youth practitioners; it is an effective way of informing government and organisational policy. It helps improve practice and can be used to challenge the many prejudicial ideas about young people that too many people take for granted. In this chapter we are mainly concerned with applied research that has an objective to transform policy, practice and wider social conditions that affect the lives of young people and their communities. As we argue here, a key way to promote good youth policy and improve practice is to *disseminate* good research. Dissemination entails communicating your ideas and findings in a persuasive fashion to the people you wish to influence. The value of dissemination, however (and the capacity for research to help bring about positive change), depends on what we mean by 'good research'.

Before you begin to think about disseminating your applied research, it is important to be sure that your research is *good*. As a first step, it is helpful to distinguish between good research and research that is unhelpful, not credible, or even damaging. As youth practitioner-researchers, it is important to be critically engaged when considering youth policy, practice and research. We would argue that just because it is called 'research', that does not mean it is good or that it can be used to support your objectives as a youth practitioner – quite the contrary. As we highlight in this chapter, a lot of poor research causes harm to young people. Given this, developing a capacity to evaluate what counts as good research is a critical skill that can make a huge different to the lives of young people, to the quality of practices and to the youth sector as a whole. In this chapter we outline key strategies to help you make this evaluation.

Once you have assessed the credibility of the research itself, you are halfway to becoming a practitioner who can 'do' and 'use' research to achieve positive change. As we suggest, dissemination requires the ability to understand how to persuade people to think or act in certain ways. This is no simple task, and there are many challenges to achieving this. For example, people are often not persuaded to change their minds or actions based on evidence alone. This is painfully obvious when you consider many serious social problems, such as climate change. Our inability to tackle climate change is in part due to people's unwillingness or inability to respond to the reams of research about the issue, and this is no less true for the many problems facing young people today. Research needs to be communicated effectively to change people's minds, feelings and actions, and this is a critical task for youth practitioners if we are serious about achieving social justice for young people. The popular belief that all we need is enough good research, filled with facts and statistics, is fallacious. If we are serious about enacting positive changes for young people, youth practitioners need to be committed to communicating good research in meaningful ways.

In this chapter, we build on these observations to identify key questions and protocols youth practitioners can use when designing and disseminating good research. First, we begin by exploring the requirements of good research. Without knowing what constitutes good research, practitioners can do a lot of damage by unwittingly disseminating bad research. Second, we go on to outline some key principles for persuasive dissemination to a broad range of audiences.

## Why good research is important: some history, ethical considerations and the myth of impartiality

### A short history of research

A helpful way to begin the task of exploring 'good research' is by focusing briefly on our historical context. This begins with the 'Age of Enlightenment' (about 1650 to the late eighteenth century) or the start of modernity or modern society, which bought about the radical new belief that 'scientific knowledge', discovered through empirical research, could free us from myth and superstition, and reveal truths about the world that could then be used to advance humanity. Indeed, the belief that scientific knowledge and research would inevitably promote human welfare, secure economic growth, and solve serious social problems continues to be a defining feature of modernity. In the popular Western imagination, research is inextricably linked to visions of social advancement and progress.

This belief is based on the assumption that we (the enlightened subjects of modernity) are rational and that we think and make decisions in reasoned, logical ways, be they in family life, career decisions or policy-making. As rational modern people who believe in the value of science, so the story goes, we are free from the interference of emotions, feelings and other 'irrational', 'primitive' sensibilities, such as superstitions or religion. By the early twentieth century, sociologists such as Max Weber (1978) were lamenting that this belief in science and the rationalisation process had led to a loss of that which had come to be seen as 'irrational', including folk magic, myth and religion. Clearly, given people's continued expression of human characteristics, such as emotions and faith, or more generally the irrational ways we think and act, this modern belief is limited. Nevertheless, it remains popular and continues to have a major influence on how we do, understand and value research.

Understanding how Western life is informed by these modern discourses about research and scientific knowledge-making is critical for appreciating the conditions in which we now live. Indeed, without this modern imaginary, science, globalisation, the economy and the welfare state in its various forms would not exist. Our faith in scientific rationality informs where and how we live, how we work and our professional identities. With modernity came new knowledge and expertise, and with that we saw the rise of a new 'professional society'. It is a context in which we witnessed not only a commitment to scientific rationality but the proliferation of 'experts' who legitimated their professional authority by claiming they had exclusive access to a unique body of knowledge (Perkin 1990). An indication of the 'normative' status of this belief is even evident in the UN's Universal Declaration on Human Rights. Article 27 declares that everyone has the right to 'share in scientific advancement and [its] benefits' (UN 1948).

## Some ethics behind research

Given the power of this narrative about our rationality and how scientific research will advance humankind, it is useful to recall the reason for the enactment of the Universal Declaration on Human Rights. The decade prior to the Universal Declaration witnessed wholesale murder on a grand scale, with large numbers of people subjected to homicidal experiments in the name of science and advancing 'the human race'. After 1945 and the end of the Second World War, the horrific nature of those experiments came to light and a number of eminent medical practitioners and scientists were placed on trial. Some were sentenced to death while others were imprisoned for war crimes because of the inhumane scientific experiments they conducted on prisoners. Those trials led to the drafting of the Nuremberg Code, a document that details the principles governing experiments on humans.

The Nuremberg Code provided a starting point for subsequent ethical codes governing research involving people and animals. The question, however, is whether such interventions have helped guarantee that research and its application are ethical. Have such codes meant that all subsequent scientific research has been ethical? The answer, clearly, is no. In the decades following the drafting of the Nuremberg Code, many hospital patients, children in institutions and prisoners were used in horrendous experiments. For example, the Tuskegee Syphilis Experiment continued until 1972 and saw 'scientists' researching the effects of untreated syphilis by withholding penicillin from 400 infected African-American crop pickers and actively ensuring that they knew nothing about their infection. As a result, 128 men died unnecessarily, 40 women (their wives) were infected and 19 children were born with congenital syphilis (Jones 1981). Issues of ethics in research are still highly contentious, as highlighted by the debates about the continued practice of animal research in the medical and cosmetic industries internationally, and the questionable ethics of killing and inflicting suffering on huge numbers of animals for such purposes.

While these may be extreme examples, they do serve to highlight that, in order to be good research, the investigative project that produces it needs to be ethical. To ensure this happens, youth practitioners need to be critically reflective about the ethical implications of their research. Solely relying on the practice of 'ticking the boxes' in prescriptive 'codes of ethics' and regulations is not enough.

## Some values behind research

'Good' research relies on the researcher, or the person using the research, being aware of the ethics and values that informed it. The stereotype of 'impartiality', where researchers do not have an interest or personal stake in their work, is a myth about science that can be quite damaging. As Gould (1981: 36) observes, the popular idea that impartiality can be achieved and that it can ensure dispassionate objectivity is misleading:

> Impartiality (even if desirable) is unattainable by human beings with inevitable backgrounds needs, beliefs and desires. It is dangerous for [a scholar to believe they can have] complete neutrality, for then one stops being vigilant about personal preferences and their influences – and then one truly falls victim to the dictates of prejudice.

We do need to be careful about claims of objectivity, because all we can ever do is be fair in the treatment of the research material. We cannot pretend to have no interests or preferences, and, as Gould (1981: 37) argues, the best way to be fair lies in recognising what our interests and preferences are so that their influence can be known and countered.

In short, to safeguard the credibility of the project, it is important to be clear to others and ourselves about our politics and interests. If we have a clear position on a subject, this means acknowledging our positionality, and being able to say, for example, that

> I am a progressive (or a conservative or an environmentalist) and proud of it, or that my research about young people . . . affirm[s] my politics. I recognise this and that recognition is helpful because it provides me with a better chance of being fair in my own work. It allows me for example to be on my guard when I develop research questions, when I collect and analyse my material. It allows the practitioner to say, I am a progressive for sound reasons, and I believe that what I report in my research is what is actually happening, and that my arguments provide information and ideas about the best ways governments and other interested parties can respond to the issues I have addressed.
>
> (Gould 1981: 37–38)

The message is simple. Whilst social researchers may claim that they are impartial or that their research is based on rational and reasoned thinking and action, and rejection of emotions or religion, we should read such claims as a warning sign. The best we can do as critically reflective researchers is to treat the material fairly; in order to do that, we must acknowledge what our own interests are. As Becker (1993: 237) put it: 'the question is not whether we should take sides, since we inevitably will, but rather whose side are we on?' Being transparent about one's positionality lends substantial credibility to your research.

# Good research

Evaluating research to determine whether it is credible involves identifying the assumptions and values that inform it. This needs to be done before dissemination; otherwise, we run the risk of distributing material that could be prejudicial and this might have serious consequences for young people and their lives.

This raises the question: what counts as good research? As was argued above, following a well-used scientific methodology or an ethical code is not enough. Given that the question of what counts as good research has been the topic of debate for centuries and that there are many different kinds of research, each with their own standards and rules, we limit our account to a few key pointers that will hopefully serve as a rough guide.

## *Defining good research: some basic criteria*

While explaining what constitutes 'good research' is relevant to this chapter, it is also a huge task. And, given our space constraints, we refer to the work of writers like Nussbaum (2000) and Sen (2009) to point us in the right direction. Drawing on their work, we argue that good research is that which enhances our capacity to exercise substantive freedom to choose to be and do what we value, and then to be resourced so we can achieve what we value (Sen 2009). For philosophers such as Nussbaum and Sen, this takes us some way towards creating a just society or a just institution in which the dignity of all is preserved.

At a basic level, we argue that good research is that which helps provide the 'social goods' needed for a good life. That is, the 'good' in 'good research' points to a plurality of social goods that have many different theoretical and practical dimensions. These can include the ability to live a healthy life free of unnecessary pain, to enjoy meaningful social relations, to pursue philosophical insight, truths or spirituality, to question what is right and to play and recreate. There are various arguments about the different kinds of social goods that enjoy widespread support from many writers across (see, for example, Finnis 1980; Sen 2009; Nussbaum 1995). 'Good research' will therefore support the realisation of some acknowledged 'social good'. Before you consider disseminating your research, it might be helpful to articulate which social goods it might support.

Not all 'scientific research' is good, and unfortunately a lot of bad research is disseminated very effectively. Young people are all too often the research targets for suspect science. The eugenic 'racial hygiene movement' that took off in the twentieth century is an example of suspect, value-laden research masquerading as neutral science. Sadly, it had a major influence of the lives of young people and on professional practice.

Racial hygiene was a 'science' that relied on racially prejudiced assumptions, including the idea that the white race was superior to all other races and that the supremacy of the British Empire could be secured by selective breeding programmes and other interventions. To ensure the British race flourished, programmes were 'needed' to discourage and encourage particular groups to reproduce, and young people were seen as the critical site of intervention. As the most fertile age in society, it was young people's reproductive capacities that were 'altered' in order to achieve the desired eugenic breeding effect. With little variation, young women of 'undesirable' status were systematically discouraged from having children – be they working class, of 'mixed race', disabled, judged to be delinquent or any other 'inferior' category. The simple belief was that through scientific control of the population, the government could engineer a more efficient, healthy and superior society for the future. Just as youth workers are now called on to help prevent unwanted teen pregnancies, they played a critical role in delivering these programmes for much of the first half of the twentieth century.

During this period, 'racial hygiene' research was at the forefront of a comprehensive movement for the promotion of scientific and rational administration of the state with a view to ensuring 'national efficiency'. Young people played a central role in this agenda. It was seen as objective science, and did not critique or explore the values underpinning its agenda. Its claims to scientific neutrality spared its prejudice from critique. Right until the 1940s, eugenics was a vanguard of 'properly constituted' scientific research. It came with a simple and profound optimism about the role of science in social progress and the important place of young people in that political imaginary. In the USA, Australia and Britain eugenics-inspired research was so effectively communicated that it led to what, in retrospect, seem extreme policies and practices, such as the sterilisation of many young people, including those with disabilities, and the use of clitoridectomies to 'prevent' girls identified as 'wayward or precocious' from becoming 'promiscuous'.

Despite the discrediting of eugenics as a science and a movement, many of its key values and intellectual practices continue in contemporary youth work, albeit without the title of eugenics itself. In Australia, for example, the Racial

Hygiene Association simply rebranded itself as the Family Planning Association in the 1960s and continued with its eugenicist commitment to prevent unnecessary and unwanted pregnancies. It remains one of the largest providers of sexual health services in the country. The eugenics discourse spoke (and its modern reincarnations still speak) with natural scientific authority about sexuality and sex, education, fertility and demography, the biological and measurable characteristics of intelligence and the role of all that in determining social and economic outcomes. 'Unhygienic' factors, such as poor education, feeble-minded children, neglected children, poor nutrition and delinquency, which diminish humankind's capacity, are problematised, underpinning a modern drive to seek scientific solutions.

---

Given that research is a project-in-time, its temporal character needs to be acknowledged. Thus, one way of talking about good research is to distinguish between the *intentions*, *processes* and *consequences* of the research project. This allows us, at least analytically, to distinguish between good (or bad) intentions, the quality of the processes and the consequences of the research, which may be either good or bad, or may have benefits or disadvantages for different people. Below, we begin to unpack ways of interrogating the intentions, processes and potential consequences that mark 'good' social research and will support the practitioner-researcher in ultimately disseminating their findings.

## Intentions

- Was there a good rationale for the research? For example, were there defensible ethical political, methodological or social reasons for doing it?

## Processes

- Was the research credible? Was it, for example, based on reliable, good-quality evidence? Was that evidence used to address the research questions or to substantiate the claims or arguments made?
- Does the research combine self-knowledge with the knowledge of the people under study, so both the researcher and the audience learn things about themselves as they/we learn about the people being researched?
- Was it methodologically sound? For example, was any research material selected and represented in ways that undermined the research process or the 'findings'?
- Were the findings presented in an open and honest way, or were they designed to manipulate the reader? For example, were impressive tables, numbers and statistical equations used in ways that invited the reader to believe that the conclusion is more certain than it actually is?
- Were the means used to achieve the research outcomes ethical?

## *Consequences*

- Did the research produce benefits that extended beyond the academy? If so, who benefited?
- Did the research identify, protect or support definable social goods?
- Who is likely to gain as a result of the research and who is likely to lose? Whose interests were served by the research? Were those interests universal or generalised interests or were they more particularistic or parochial?
- Were the research findings acceptable and understandable to the people who were studied? In other words, was it close to how those being studied would interpret their values, experiences and actions? Or was it overly generalised, abstract and unrecognisable to those being studied?
- Does the research make a positive contribution to the existing body of knowledge and 'truth'?
- Was the research informed by explicit ethical goods embedded in the research questions/design? For instance, when designing the research, were specific goods identified explicitly in the research design?

While this is not an exhaustive list of criteria, hopefully it provides a general guide for identifying good research.

# Research and the task of interpreting it

How research is interpreted matters. We can have research that is scientifically credible, generated in ethical ways, with clearly articulated values and supportive of clear social good, but it might be interpreted in ways that are unhelpful, not sensible, and possibly even damaging.

What we are talking about is the distinction between research and how it is interpreted and used. To illustrate, we need only refer to the latest neurological research that used non-invasive brain-scan technology to 'discover' that the 'adolescent brain' matures later than we originally thought. This research was been picked up by many non-experts in neurology and interpreted in ways that justify common prejudices that young people are 'hard-wired for risk' (Bessant 2008: 347–360). In other words, it may not be the research itself that is problematic, but how it is interpreted and used. In this case, we saw some 'youth experts' interpreting results from the 'adolescent brain research' that revealed changes to nerve growth in young people up to the age of twenty-five and using it to reinforce negative stereotypes. This led to erroneous conclusions that science was confirming what we already suspected: 'Adolescents . . . are crazy according to a primal blueprint; they are crazy by design' (Straunch 2004: xiv). In this instance, scientific results were interpreted in ways that were deeply problematic, and they were used to argue for policy reforms and changes to practice that negatively impact on young people (Bessant 2008).

This is an example of how good research can be interpreted in ways that do not enhance the well-being of young people or the community. In the case of 'adolescent brain science', good neurological research is being interpreted in ways that might affirm ageist prejudices about young people, and it is used to describe or frame 'youth' in ways that encourage regressive responses. If being irresponsible is biologically determined, then 'we' should limit 'their' rights and opportunities. If the research that reveals certain changes are taking place in the brains of young people is interpreted to mean young people are inherently biologically wired to be reckless and unable to make good judgements, which causes them to be delinquent, criminal and accident prone, then the solution is that new, restrictive laws and policies are needed to address that problem. This is an example of how effective dissemination of good research that has been interpreted in problematic ways can influence legislation dealing with everything from the age of criminal culpability to education, to say nothing of its impact on institutional policy and professional practices, and indeed the very experience of being young.

What all this means is that 'good research' includes more than whether it conforms to basic methodological conventions. It also needs to be ethical and support 'social goods'. And it must be interpreted in ways that, at the very least, do not cause harm and, ideally, enhance the lives of young people. Ensuring that good research is disseminated and used requires the practitioner to have a capacity to spot work that is unethical, not credible, or prejudice masquerading as science.

What we are saying is that compliance with the conventional rules of science (the so-called 'scientific method' entails identifying a question, constructing a hypothesis, testing the hypothesis through data collection, analysing and interpreting the data, and drawing conclusions) does not necessarily guarantee good research. Given the authority that scientific research has enjoyed amongst people in the youth sector, and the general public, this may be a little disconcerting for some people. Why do social researchers disagree so much about youth issues? The answer is that we see and interpret youth problems differently because researchers operate with different assumptions, different ethical ideas and different understandings of the nature of reality and how social reality can be accessed or known. Some social researchers subscribe to the idea that social reality is somehow 'out there', simply waiting to be discovered and reported on, and that this reality can be accessed through 'scientific means'. Others suggest it is not so simple. The differences in these ways of seeing are reflected in the philosophical traditions that have informed research over the centuries. Knowing something about them is important for being able to determine what counts contextually as 'good research'. For the sake of simplicity, we identify two key social science traditions that have informed research and knowledge-making practices. The first is the empirical positivist tradition and the second the interpretivist or hermeneutic tradition.

Within the conventional empirical tradition, the authority of 'science' rests on a popular belief that 'scientific methods' provide a clear set of rules that researchers simply follow. If they apply them correctly, the result will be 'good science'. But is this true? Those methods include careful use of empirical observation, measurement, fact finding, preferably the use of statistics that are replicable, and disciplined objectivity, which prohibits emotion, sectional interests or values. Doing research in this way is said to give scientists an ability to reveal underlying laws or patterns and theoretical ideas, and gives them the ability to provide explanations and make predictions. From Galileo's and Newton's research on physics, to the later social research by Durkheim and Merton, the recurring assumption has been that obedience to the protocols of science guarantees good science, which then simply needs to be communicated and applied to fix social problems.

The second philosophical tradition highlights the value of youth workers thinking critically and being informed about the key research traditions. The interpretivist or hermeneutic tradition offers an alternative to the conventional approach that is particularly valuable for those interested in understanding the human condition. It suggests that 'scientific methods' do not offer the best way of understanding social life, and that 'data' or 'facts' in science too often rely on unspoken prejudices about quite central issues, such as what counts as 'a fact'. According to Holton (1988), for example, all science relies on assumptions or 'themata'. For youth work, this is a helpful insight because much of the research on young people has, arguably, been informed by prejudicial assumptions (Gould 1981).

Equally subversive and important for youth workers is the argument that science is a social practice where the most powerful typically have a say in what truth is, and in what counts as real. Issues of power and knowledge are especially pertinent here. Given that young people tend to have less power relative to other age cohorts (consider, for example, the age restrictions on political representation, and legal and financial autonomy), this is significant. Our knowledge reflects the ability of the powerful to define it. Given also that young people themselves are rarely involved in knowledge-making processes generally and knowledge-making about 'youth' in particular, this insight is likely to have considerable resonance for youth work. Knowledge-making – claims to name what is true and have others accept that as truth – is an exercise of power in which young people typically lose out because they tend not to get a say. The history of knowledge-making *about* young people is littered with examples of damaging assumptions relating to 'the nature of youth'.

Philosophers and post-structuralists such as Foucault (1976), as well as discourse analysts like Fairclough (1992), claim that the findings of research – 'truths' – comprise a language game, and that the notion of 'truth' is socially constructed to conform with what powerful people determine it to be. In this way 'truth' is not so much the result of rigorous scientific research but rather an effect of power.

These cautionary tales are now the basis of rich and diverse philosophical debates. However, while these may be fascinating, it is not our intention to expand on them here. Rather, our priority is to explore the strategies that can be deployed to disseminate good research and to persuade the potential audiences of the value of your social research. Before addressing this, though, it was important to explore what conventionally counts as good research processes, the credibility of research values, how good research can result in potentially bad outcomes, and finally to query the conventional wisdom about scientific methods and social progress. All of these issues raise questions about how we interpret and judge what is happening around us and how people might be persuaded to change their minds and actions by research. This is key to understanding effective dissemination, to which we now turn.

## Effective dissemination, persuading people and communicating ideas

Despite the modern Western, near-hegemonic belief in objectivity and scientific ratio-nality, decades of research by psychologists and communications researchers have demonstrated that research findings have relatively little sway in influencing what people actually believe. This is partly because people generally do not like to hear views that contrast with their own, or to have to accommodate views that are too different, ideas or facts that challenge what they already know, think and feel. Psychologists refer to 'cognitive dissonance' to describe what happens when people keep a belief or make a claim to know something when there is clear evidence to the contrary. A recent example of this is sceptics' dogged insistence that we do not face an environmental global-warming problem and that there is no need to reduce carbon emissions.

We tend to be persuaded by facts and stories that affirm what we already 'know' or feel. It is easy to persuade people about things that reinforce their existing worldview. When we talk about worldviews and popular assumptions about young people, they are typically prejudicial and imagine 'youth' as troubled and troublesome. So research that produces 'findings' to the contrary tends to attract little interest. New scientific ideas that challenge conventional wisdom, even if they are supported by theoretical or empir-ical data, are often resisted by those loyal to older paradigms. Obvious examples, such as Galileo's attempts to convince the Catholic Church that the world was not flat, litter our history.

According to cognitive scientists, such as George Lakoff (1999; Lakoff and Johnson 2003), if we plan to change people's minds, then we need to do more than present scien-tific research and facts. We also need to pay attention to the techniques entailed in reframing debates. This does not mean throwing out the 'rational evidence model' of social research, but rather looking more closely at how language is used in communicating ideas about research. Lakoff enquired into the ways people think by exploring, pertinently for us, public policy discourses in the United States. His work is germane to our task because he invites us to confront certain popular myths about human knowledge and thinking. He also pays particular attention to metaphors and how they influence thinking, and how our values and feelings rely on the ways we think and make judgements.

In his case study, Lakoff argues that the ascendancy of conservatism in America's policy-making communities over the past three decades can largely be credited to effective communication on behalf of conservative advocates. These people were, until recently, able to construct more authoritative, emotional and ethically appealing poli-tics. Their success was not achieved because they had better or more credible research on which to draw. Conservative advocates made particular use of metaphors to connect certain ideas with values and feelings that were deeply ingrained and very popular in the USA. They recognised the political value of identifying and tapping into the views, ideas and feelings of large numbers of people, whilst many progressives dismissed these as irrational, silly and unworthy. Lakoff (2005) recognised the strategies used by the right – specifically how they connected widely shared emotions, values and prejudices to develop convincing, albeit largely fictitious, images of the world. By doing this, conservatives were very successful in framing the country's social problems in ways that persuaded many people that they were 'caused' by too many violent teenage thugs, drugged-up party wasters, work-shy young people and spiralling numbers of welfare-dependent single mothers spawning children to jump the housing queue, all of whom were contributing to a state of general decline. Furthermore, this was happening at the expense of 'us' – responsible, adult, hard-working taxpayers who were disciplined and self-reliant.

Similar communication strategies have played out in much the same way in the UK. The appeal to shared emotions, values and prejudices was on full display when the Conservative Social Security Secretary Peter Lilley burst into song at the 1992 Tory Party conference, crooning:

> I've got a little list
> Of benefit offenders who I'll soon be rooting out
> And who never would be missed . . .
> Young ladies who get pregnant to jump the housing list
> And the dads who won't support the children of the ladies they have kissed
> And I haven't even mentioned those sponging Socialists
> I've got them on my list
> And there's none of them be missed.

Mnemonic communication at its finest; youth practitioners take note. The contemporary rise of the debate about 'Broken Britain' shares much with this narrative.

Lakoff makes the helpful observation that the immediate response of 'the left' or 'progressives' was to critique their opponents. While criticism is important, it is also potentially damaging because it allows 'the other side' to establish the terms of the debate. Rebutting a negative frame can evoke and reinforce that frame in people's minds, because it encourages the listener to imagine what we are critiquing rather than what we are proposing. For example, if you are told not to think of an elephant, you will almost certainly think about an elephant. The lesson here, for those for interested in youth advocacy, is that when we produce research findings that say young people are not irresponsible, lazy hoodies, we need to be careful that we are not evoking the negative images we are criticising. In short, when we advocate for or with young people by denying such stereotypes, we can buy into those negative framings, and thereby invite the audience to see young people as troubled and troublesome. Instead, we need to present a much more positive framing of young people.

According to Lakoff, the conservative movement was successful because they understood how people think and how to reach out to win their support. The left, on the other hand, focused too much on critiquing the right and not enough on constructing alternative and appealing ideas, values and metaphors to frame their own policies.

In short, understanding how research can be used to persuade audiences is vital, but that understanding needs to be informed by a capacity to determine whether research is good.

Once we have the research in hand and have exercised due diligence in checking it is good, what next? How do we communicate it and persuade others of its worth? Given that people tend to be resistant to facts that do not support what they already believe, there can be obstacles to persuading others. We argue here that persuading people of the validity of a particular point of view requires a positive frame that appeals to their feelings and values and uses appropriate metaphors to carry the desired message. With this in mind, we now turn to the question of *how* to disseminate.

## The need for effective dissemination in youth practice

The conventional belief that research is conducted only in universities by highly qualified researchers and postgraduate students is a very partial view. Some of the best youth research has been done outside of academia by busy youth practitioners. It takes many different forms, ranging from needs assessments to community profiles. As this can form a substantive component of youth practice, it is vital that practitioners make the most of their hard work and communicate their ideas to appropriate audiences.

Typically, most people conduct research to 'discover' new things or to generate new products, new ideas or new ways of seeing. While some people may research for pleasure, most social researchers enquire into social problems to try to effect change in some way. It may be research intended to discover the needs of young people in a particular community which can then be used as evidence to support a bid for new services, or it may be research that challenges what is seen as a discriminatory practice. As the Danish social scientist Bjent Flyvbjerg (2001) argued, good research generates positive change. Youth-focused research of this kind would be research that tackles problems that matter to young people. Sometimes the purpose of youth research is to clarify, sometimes to intervene, sometimes to generate new perspectives. Its purpose is always to assist in an ongoing effort to generate better understanding of the lives of young people and the contexts in which they live, and to shape a future in which they can develop as best they can (Flyvbjerg 2001: 166). Given this, good youth research is lost without a thoughtful dissemination strategy.

Actively sharing research findings and results is part of a larger democratisation of knowledge. Spreading research-based ideas helps to ensure that as many people as possible can put the knowledge generated through research to good use. Youth practitioners are obliged to share their specialist knowledge and expertise with the communities in which young people live, with a view to improving their lives. Research can play a role in the development of youth work only if it is complemented by a thoughtful approach to persuading people.

The role of practitioners who work with young people is to help them develop a voice in various public spheres and an influence within their community. As the National Occupational Standards for Youth Work in the UK suggests, this rests on our ability to help educate communities in ways that encourage receptiveness to the needs and aspirations of young people. This educative role relies in large part on a willingness and ability to share knowledge that will help members of 'the community' better understand the lives and experiences of young people. In short, disseminating good research about, with or for young people is a core part of good professional practice.

Given the prevalence of prejudices and stereotypes about young people – from being troubled and troublesome 'hoodies' to vulnerable children who need 'saving' – this educative role is important. Many people claim to 'know for a fact' that all young people like to get into fights and that their brains make them behave in irresponsible ways. What better way to challenge such misconceptions than by presenting your own research?

Research conducted by youth practitioners can benefit young people and their communities. In this way, it can be seen as a form of advocacy, and the dissemination of good research is a key role for practitioners who work with young people.

## Key issues in dissemination

As we are concerned with applied research in this chapter, it is important to point out that the end point of your work as a youth researcher is not printing off the final copy of your research report and putting it on the shelf. You must still turn that report into action. To give youth research life and bring about the change you desire, the results need to be communicated. Getting your research 'out there' is called dissemination. It entails sharing or broadcasting your ideas or findings to a wide audience – your peers, the community and young people themselves (Welch-Ross and Fasig 2007: 2).

Doing this well demands the development of a thoughtful plan. It requires more than simply publishing your results (in practice or academic journals, for example) and hoping they somehow get 'picked up'. It is easy to fall into the trap of thinking that communicating your research with a selected audience means it will somehow translate magically and effortlessly into appropriate responses (McCall and Groark 2007). Dissemination is more than reporting or describing what you did and what you discovered. It is a strategic and targeted process that provides opportunities to turn your findings into action. It is an opportunity that can have results if you appreciate the value of understanding the context in which you are operating.

Gary Marx (1997: 115) suggests that social researchers should be as active as possible in the dissemination process and should seek to get as much 'leverage' out of their work as they can. You could, for example, turn your research into professional development for colleagues or students, publish it in a journal article, reprint it in books, post it on blogs, or use it to inform a documentary or your work with policy-makers. In short, think as widely as you can about dissemination and use as many means as possible.

Given the potential scope of this dissemination project, it is wise to think about it as early as possible. If your aim is to maximise your leverage and influence, then it is helpful to keep this end part of the research project in mind at each stage, from the initial design to data collection and final write-up. When you select your research topic, a clear understanding of why the problem or topic is being addressed helps. While collecting your data, ask what cases or types of evidence will be most effective in helping you communicate with and persuade your audience(s). If, for example, you want to convince hard-nosed economists, then it will be prudent to include some traditional empirical data or statistics. If you want to help the audience understand a problem like student poverty, then you may need to include ethnographic evidence or insider accounts so your audience has access to clear narratives about what financial hardship means in everyday life. So, think strategically and plan in advance. In terms of developing a strategy, the following six questions might be useful prompts for reflection (based on Welch-Ross and Fasig 2007: 5).

## What should be disseminated?

As discussed above, before you even think about dissemination it is helpful to reflect on what you are hoping to communicate and change. Only good research that is presented well is likely to lead to positive outcomes for young people. If your research does not meet the criteria to be considered 'good' research, then do not disseminate it.

## Who is your audience?

Select your audience strategically. Think about dissemination as you do your research, so by the time you are ready to disseminate it, you will have a fairly clear idea about the changes you would like to see. You may, for example, have captured the impact of a bad practice at a local health clinic, or the success of a great local scheme that you think should be rolled out further. Think about to whom you will show your research to have the kind of influence you desire, and identify who can help make your change happen – they are your key audience.

Your message also needs to match your audience. Different audiences require different styles of communication, different pitches, language and formats. Communicating effectively can also depend on your ability to convey complex ideas and material in ways that are convincing. How this is done varies according to the audience. If the task is to persuade a person or a group about ideas or findings based on your research, then you will need to do a little research on your audience.

Some background information on the people you want to influence is critical. What are their experiences and attitudes towards the issue in question? What are their formal and informal positions? Being context sensitive rests on knowing something of the people you are communicating with, as well as something of the institution and the broader social or political context in which they operate. It entails asking what cultural and institutional practices or beliefs are likely to have a bearing on your argument. For example, if the addressee works in a children's court or a local council, then institutional requirements, rules and laws will influence how you present your material. In the same way, quite specific customs or protocols (including courtesies) operate in many communities. If the people you are working with belong to a religious or ethnic community, particular dress codes and other rules about the body may apply. These context-specific nuances are especially important.

Strauss and Corbin (1990) have identified four general audiences for social science research: academics, policy-makers, practitioners and the general public. While these are very broad categories, they offer a guide. It may help you anticipate their different expectations that will inform your style and pitch, and how you frame the problem your research addresses.

## Academics

Writing for an academic audience typically entails complying with particular conventions that vary according to discipline area. This can make effective communication difficult, as practitioners may not have the patience or the time to learn these protocols. Co-authoring with an academic is a sensible option because it draws on the expertise you may not have in reaching another audience.

In terms of format, presentations at academic conferences are one convention. These involve researchers sharing their findings and ideas in conference workshops with other academics and practitioners. This would usually involve a PowerPoint presentation that outlines your research question, theory, methodology and findings. The academy also values academic texts highly, so publishing your research findings in academic journals or as book chapters is always a good idea.

## Policy-makers

'Policy-makers' is a general category that includes those who work within the 'inner sanctum' of government or an organisation where decisions are made, as well as people working in broader networks and groups that influence policy-making (e.g. how a youth problem is constituted and addressed). The policy-making community might include civil servants, members of government at the local, regional and national levels, journalists, funding agencies, youth advocacy groups and NGOs. They are 'idealised' targets for social researchers, with an interest in 'practical information'. They tend to look for material and ideas that are relevant to current policy agendas, and are generally unreceptive to big change ideas.

According to Hadley (1987), researchers often complain about 'not being heard' by policy-makers. This, he says, may be due to the nature of the research itself, for three key reasons:

1   Research is sometimes commissioned to buy time to address 'moral panics' that flare up in the political realm. An inquiry called into X or Y might not be valued for the results it produces, but rather because it allows policy-makers to use it to appease critics and 'an angry public' and to demonstrate that 'something is being done'.
2   The time taken to produce quality research often means that political priorities have shifted by the time findings are disseminated, and thus policy-makers lose interest because the issue is seen to be outdated.
3   Researchers are easily dismissed as idealistic, out of touch or unrealistic when they deliver politically undesirable findings (Hadley 1987: 100–102).

While attracting the attention of policy-makers can be difficult, this does not mean the task should be abandoned. The following advice may help you to communicate effectively with policy-makers.

•   Frame your research in acceptable language. Political issues and policy problems are often fashionable. They tend to address concerns that emerge as trends, and are often reactions to public opinion. With this in mind, we suggest that you consider whether your research can be framed in a way to demonstrate its relevance to current trends or issues. Survey the prevailing policy issues.

- Is there an event, such as the International Year of the Young Person or the anniversary of the Convention on the Rights of the Child, that might lend your findings some popular appeal?
- Produce clear and succinct findings and recommendations from your research and have a clear message. While the findings from your research will inevitably be complex, and God is in the detail of your work, policy-makers are busy people. Identifying a concise set of recommendations and easy-to-understand messages will improve your chances of being heard.

In terms of format, reaching policy-makers requires a context-specific approach. You also need to identify who might be interested in the kind of change you have in mind, and who has the power or capacity to make such a change. The next step is to identify how you can communicate with those people and which channels are open to you.

## Practitioners

While some practitioners look for a theoretical framework that will help them better understand their clients, their workplace and the contexts in which they work, others are dismissive of theory, arguing that it is irrelevant and that all they need are the 'straight facts', models or applicable solutions to 'real, on-the-ground problems'.

There is clearly a tension here that you need to acknowledge and consider when disseminating your research. If you want to highlight theoretical insights that can benefit practice, make sure you explain their relevance clearly. Likewise, when delivering 'empirical' findings, it may be useful to challenge the myth that 'facts' or 'empirical research' can ever be theory free. Research that is seen to have immediate 'practical application' and provides insight into problems faced in practitioners' day-to-day work are likely to have appeal.

In terms of format, information can be shared with practitioners in print through practitioner journals or popular professional blogs and magazines (*Children and Young People Now*, for example), or in person at networking events (such as the Federation for Detached Youth Workers' annual conference and other local and national youth work events). If you are a practitioner yourself, think about where you go to receive information. How do you like to hear about new ideas? Obviously, you are a great source of knowledge about practitioners such as yourself!

## The general public

We have already talked about the value of democratising knowledge, and sharing your findings as broadly as possible includes the wider public. According to Silverman (2006), there are good reasons for disseminating your research to the general public:

- Sharing your findings with the community and young people, especially if they were involved in the project itself, gives them the chance to hear the results. It also gives them a chance to discover what is happening in their community, something that may have an educative value and can also enhance community relations.

- Sharing preliminary findings as you are still analysing and concretising your ideas can provide a valuable 'reality check'. This is particularly important if you are drawing on the community as a source of research material. It can help ensure that participants within the community are happy with the ways they are represented and that their voices are not being usurped by the researcher.

However, communication with 'the public' can be tricky. To explain what we mean by 'public', we point to spaces where 'citizens' discuss public issues or criticise arbitrary and unreasonable authority and power (Habermas 1968). The 'public sphere' is seen to be central to all modern democracies and is described as a space where criticism and discussions about public matters, such as rights (e.g. to assemble freely, to elect governments and to criticise them) and freedoms (of speech, information and so on), are encouraged. All this helps form what has come to be known as 'public opinion'. 'Public' also refers to events, processes and places that are not closed or exclusive affairs. (Having said that, we acknowledge that in spite of the assumption that 'public' means 'open to all', young people are often excluded from 'the public sphere'.)

In terms of a communication strategy, basic public relations practices suggest that you narrow down your audience to a target cohort. It could be people living in a particular neighbourhood, or mothers who should be using a particular service. Not even the biggest brands, with huge budgets and popular appeal, try to target the whole population with one message. Think how each campaign can be strategically devised to appeal to one particular sector or segment of the public. Identify your target groups and tailor your message accordingly. The format you choose will again depend on your audience.

## Who should disseminate the research?

Reflect on which messages you can deliver yourself, and which others might be better suited to deliver. We have already discussed the option of co-authoring with an academic if you are seeking to influence academics. Likewise, collaborating with NGOs or grassroots networks can make your arguments more persuasive. Often it is more effective, and better for other reasons, if young people 'spread the word' themselves, especially if your target audience is other young people. Take a moment to reflect on who might be able to assist you in this. With whom can you collaborate for your dissemination to add weight to your arguments?

## When should you disseminate the research?

The timeliness of a research-inspired intervention can be critical. Issuing a press release on your latest research at the right time can make a big difference in terms of the reception you receive and its impact. If your research relates to specific political and policy issues, then, as mentioned earlier, it may help to remember how such 'issues' can be fashionable at particular times. If, however, you are working in an area like youth homelessness, then it is likely there will always be interest because it is a perennial problem. The same can be said of research in other persistently problematic domains, such as child protection. Reflect on the best time for the dissemination of your research.

Does your research connect to a current trend or issue? If not, can you relate it to topical issues of the day? Is there an upcoming event on which you can 'piggy-back', such as the International Year of the Young Person? Can you 'link up' to gain an audience and allow them to see how your work connects to something in which people are already interested? All of these add timely persuasion to your arguments.

## How can the research be communicated?

Once you have selected an audience, a format and a time, you need to think about how to deliver your findings. Are they, for example, best communicated through a policy briefing, as professional development for practitioners, or through articles in the press? What options do you have, and what will deliver the 'best bang for your buck'?

This is where working out what frame you will use becomes critical. As Lakoff (2005) suggests, if you are interested in persuading others, then it helps to use a positive frame that connects with the people you are trying to influence. To get this right, you might run some focus groups or do some homework to establish what your target audience already believes and knows, how they feel and what they value.

You also need to think about the language that you will use and how you might employ certain metaphors. Can you make changes, through metaphors, that encourage your audience to see you and your work in a more positive light?

The sixth and final question is the most important.

## What do you wish to achieve?

What actions or changes would you like to see as a result of your intervention? Try to be specific about the changes you want to see. If you cannot succinctly summarise your findings into bullet-point recommendations, you cannot expect your audience to make this translation. You need to be very clear about what you want to happen as a result of your research. Present your findings clearly and concisely as achievable recommendations if you want to see change.

Before disseminating any research, you need to determine whether it deserves to be disseminated. This requires an ability to produce good research or a capacity to think critically about the work of others that you plan to disseminate or use to inform your own practice.

Producing good research and communicating it effectively require a clear understanding of the socio-political context in which you are working. Youth researchers have much to gain from recognising how they can tune into the politics of their immediate milieu and broader context in ways that advance the interests of young people. In short, your capacity to effect change by producing and communicating research is likely to increase if you are mindful of your socio-political context. The question is how you can make your research work for young people.

Like any social science, good youth research is done, as Flyvbjerg (2001: 166), says, 'in public for the public, sometimes to clarify, sometimes to intervene, sometimes to generate new perspectives, and always to serve as the eyes and ears in our on-going efforts at understanding the present and deliberating about the future'. In short, good youth research is wasted without a clear action plan that spells out how it can be disseminated in ways that will bring about desired changes.

## Practice-based task 9.1  Developing a dissemination strategy

Using your current research project, follow this schedule to develop a dissemination strategy.

### Before dissemination

- Is your research 'fair'? Y/N (If no, do not continue)
- Was your research ethical? Y/N (If no, do not continue)
- What social good does your research support? (If you cannot identify at least one, do not continue)
- Is your research likely to produce 'positive changes'? Y/N (If no, do not continue)
- Might your research make things worse? Y/N (If yes, do not continue)

### To develop your dissemination strategy

- What changes do you want to see as a result of your research?
- What are your clear and succinct recommendations?
- Who has the 'power' to make these changes? That is, who are your audiences?
- What factors might be important to consider when communicating with your audiences? (Who funds them, what are there politics etc.?)
- How are you going to disseminate your findings?
- What 'positive frame' are you going to use to communicate your ideas to these audiences?
- When would be a good time to disseminate your findings?
- Who should you partner with to disseminate this research?
- What are you going to disseminate to these audiences?
- What format will you use (research report, articles, seminar, presentations, website, exhibition, etc.)?

## Summary of key points

We argued that before thinking about dissemination, it is critical to be able to distinguish between good and bad research. Good research is ethically produced, honest about its values, supports a social good and is generally 'helpful' for young people. To make a positive change, however, good research needs to be disseminated. Dissemination is a critical component of the research project that involves thoughtful planning about who to 'target' and how to communicate effectively. If the objective is to influence how people think, see and feel about particular issues and then act accordingly, then attention needs to be given to how we describe 'the problem'. To do this, Lakoff suggests we should pay attention to the role of metaphors and frame issues in ways that invite our audience to see things positively.

In the later part of the chapter, we identified certain steps that may work as a guide for developing a dissemination plan, with an emphasis on the importance of paying attention to your audience. This involves being context sensitive and entails (among other things) enquiry into the protocols, group dynamics, attitudes and disposition of your audience.

## Suggestions for further reading

Flyvbjerg, B. (2001) *Making Social Sciences Matter*, Cambridge: Cambridge University Press.
Welch-Ross, M. and Fasig, L. (2007) *Handbook on Communicating and Disseminating Behavioural Sciences*, London: Sage.

## References

Becker, G. (1993 [1964]) *Human Capital: A Theoretical and Empirical Analysis, with Special Reference to Education*, 3rd edn, Chicago: University of Chicago Press.
Becker, H. (1967) 'Whose Side Are We on?', *Social Problems*, 14, 239–247.
Beecher, H. (1966) 'Ethics and Clinical Research', *New England Journal of Medicine*, June, 1354–1360.
Bessant, J. (2008) 'Hard Wired for Risk: Neurological Science, the Adolescent Brain and Developmental Theory', *Journal of Youth Studies*, 11 (3), 347–360.
Fairclough, N. (1992) *Discourse and Social Change*, Cambridge: Polity Press.
Finnis, J. (1980) *Natural Law and Natural Rights*, Oxford: Oxford University Press.
Flyvbjerg, B. (2001) *Making Social Sciences Matter*, Cambridge: Cambridge University Press.
Foucault. M. (1976) *The Order of Things*, London: Hutchinson.
Gould, S.J. (1981) *The Mismeasure of Man*, London: Norton House.
Habermas, J. (1968) *Towards a Rational Society*, London: Heinemann.
Hadley, R. (1987) 'Publish and be Ignored; Proselytise and be Damned', in G. Wenger (ed.), *The Research Relationship: Practice and Politics in Social Policy*, London: Allen and Unwin, 98–110.
Holton, G. (1988) *Thematic Origins of Scientific Thought: Kepler to Einstein*, 2nd edn, New York: Harvard Univsity Press.

Jones, J. (1981) *Bad Blood: The Tuskegee Syphilis Experiment: A Tragedy of Race and Medicine*, New York: The Free Press.

Lakoff, G. (1999) *Moral Politics: How Conservatives and Liberals Think*, Chicago: University of Chicago Press.

Lakoff, G. (2005) *Don't Think of an Elephant*, Melbourne: Scribe.

Lakoff, G. and Johnson, M. (2003) *Metaphors We Live By*, Chicago: University of Chicago Press.

Marx, G. (1997) 'Of Methods and Manners for Aspiring Sociologists: 37 Moral Imperatives', *American Sociologist*, Spring, 102–125.

McCall, R.B. and Groark, C.J. (2007) 'A Perspective on the History and Future of Disseminating Behavioral and Social Science', in M.K. Welch-Ross and L.G. Fasig (eds), *Handbook on Communicating and Disseminating Behavioral Science*, Thousand Oaks, CA: Sage.

Nussbaum, M. (1995) 'Human Capabilities, Female Human Beings', in M. Nussbaum and J. Glover (eds), *Women, Culture and Development*, Oxford: Oxford University Press.

Nussbaum, M. (2000) *Women and Human Development: The Capabilities Approach*, Cambridge: Cambridge University Press.

Perkin, H. (1990) *The Rise of Professional Society*, London: Routledge.

Sen, A. (2009) *The Idea of Justice*, New York: Harvard University Press.

Silverman, D. (2006) *Interpreting Qualitative Data*, London: Sage.

Straunch, B. (2004) *The Primal Teen: What New Discoveries about the Teenage Brain Tell Us about Our Kids*, New York: Anchor Books.

Strauss, A. and Corbin, J. (1990) *Basics of Qualitative Research: Grounded Theory Procedures and Techniques*, London: Sage.

United Nations (1948) *Universal Declaration of Human Rights*, G.A. res. 217A (III), UN Doc A/810.

Weber, M. (1978) *Economy and Society: An Outline of Interpretative Sociology*, 2 vols. Berkeley, CA: UCLA Press.

Welch-Ross, M. and Fasig, L. (2007) *Handbook on Communicating and Disseminating Behavioural Sciences*, London: Sage.

<table>
<tr><td>10</td></tr>
</table>

# Research and work with young people

## Politics, participation and policy

Fin Cullen and Simon Bradford

## Overview

In Chapter 1 we explored the tensions of being both a researcher *and* a youth practitioner and we referred to the *practitioner-researcher* as a legitimate identity. In this
chapter we consider the contemporary wider political agenda that focuses on the
rhetoric of participation in youth research, policy and practice settings. The chapter
returns to a number of questions that we have explored throughout the volume. We are
particularly interested here in thinking through the impact and role of practitioner-
researcher interventions within the realms of policy, practice and theory. The majority
of this volume has concentrated on the *processes* of research, including research
methods, forms of data, dissemination and how we might ethically conduct research.

In this final chapter we consider the landscape on which contemporary debates about
youth policy and practice are located, including the role of evidence and opinion in the
construction of knowledge in policy and practice, neo-managerialist agendas and how
practitioner-researchers may contribute to the construction of knowledge and interventions in policy and practice.

Before exploring these issues in more depth, it is worthwhile exploring the current
youth policy and research terrain. One key issue that emerged in the earlier chapters is
the status of knowledge within youth research and practitioner research and the
compelling and enduring questions of what knowledge is for, and what claims we might
make for these accounts. Given that power is always implicated in the practices and
processes of knowledge production, how can we be sure that the knowledge we produce
as practitioner-researchers can stand up to scrutiny and challenge?

In the later part of this chapter we return to the contemporary youth research agenda
and the use of evidence-based practice within policy and practice debates.

## Policy and research interest in 'youth'

In recent years a burgeoning literature in childhood and youth studies has highlighted an ongoing academic interest in children and young people's social worlds and childhood and adolescence as stages in the 'life course'. Within the policy realm, the social categories of childhood and youth remain areas of great public concern. The flourishing of child and youth policy and funding for youth and education projects over the past two decades in the UK has led to a growing army of established and new children's and youth professionals tasked with tackling a range of social issues that impact on children and young people (Watts 2002; Smith 2004).

Regular moral panics erupt around the problem of troubled and troubling youth (Griffin 1993), from failing pupils to teen pregnancy, youth unemployment, knife and gun crime and street gangs (Griffin 1993; Jones 2009; Jeffs and Smith 1999). Within the policy realm, youth research is often commissioned to 'fix' perceived social ills. However, its findings risk being subsumed into governments' preconceived ideological remedies.

The 'youth' category in policy and commissioned research is discursively framed around youth as a problem invariably with the presumption that wayward young people need to be fixed by professional and policy intervention (Griffin 1993; Jeffs and Smith 1999; Jones 2009). Nearly twenty years ago, this tension was explored in depth in *Representations of Youth* (1993), in which Chris Griffin laid out a number of concerns and examined the politics of youth research in the 1980s. Much of the critique offered by Griffin still resonates in the continued discursive production of 'youth in crisis' in research, policy and practice. However, a growing body of work has acknowledged young people's active agency in challenging normative and pathologising productions of youth. As Jones (2009: 182) argues: 'The "youth question" becomes a matter of public concern. Why? One answer could be in the way young people have been seen as a social barometer, as an indicator of the state of society they live in, rather than the state of youth itself.' Jones highlights how this ongoing public interest in youth can be understood as a quest by the wider society to try to take control of the future. Similar observations have been made about the futurity of childhood (Jenks 2005).

Clearly, continuing policy concerns around the problems of youth place both practitioners and researchers in a highly contentious political arena. Children's and youth policy (including education) has been constantly reconfigured over the decades, highlighting the administrative desire to guide and shape future citizens for the good of the nation. This positions youth practitioner-researchers in a curious and interesting duality in researching *and* potentially operationalising the wider desire to repair the perceived deficiencies of youth. Armstrong (2004) argues that an industry of youth research has grown up around the policy intentions and administrations of the state, rather than contributing to wider public debates about youth policy. This is an enduring tension within the current structures, the available funding streams, and research priorities in the field of social and youth research. Administrative agencies may focus on 'curing' social ills and the indirect pathologisation of disempowered groups such as youth, rather than, for example, developing robust critiques, transformative action or new theoretical paradigms. Such tensions expand into the sphere of practitioner research, where funding and management support may be readily available only for projects that are seen to contribute to and directly support existing policy intentions, rather than wider goals focusing on transformative policy and practice and the development of usable theory.

Thus, practitioner-researchers may find themselves co-opted into roles where they need to rationalise existing and future policy and practice through their research, rather than generating new insights or taking critical responses beyond extant policy and practice assumptions. Youth practitioners, whether working in community work, education, youth work or criminal justice contexts, are precisely tasked with the 'fixing' and 'control' aspects highlighted by Jones (2009). Whether a youth practitioner-researcher chooses to focus on young people's cultures or issues of policy and practice, the ongoing policy agenda remains predicated on the broad 'youth question'.

## Reconsidering social research, policy and practice

Social research and professional work with young people are both fundamentally *political* activities. In considering the nature of the political within social research, Hammersley (2001) mobilises this through exploring questions of power and the values contained within the research. Thus, youth research and youth practice are shaped by the outcomes that are deemed contextually and situationally valuable by various funding regimes and policy priorities. As with other forms of social policy, a growing interest in youth research necessitates an active engagement from youth workers (and here one might also include other children's and youth practitioners). In the UK in recent years debates have raged over the need for youth and children's services to be accountable, cost effective and of clear use to wider society in educating and supporting young people for a variety of different political agendas. Similar battles have raged over the nature, quality and impact of social research within research councils and other research organisations.

Here, it is important to note the importance of the *goal* of social research. Should it be about the 'production of knowledge' (Hammersley 1995: 118)? In a paper exploring the purpose of social research in addressing social problems, Bloor (1997) considers whether researchers should focus on influencing policy-makers or practitioners. Bloor highlights that early sociological work considered approaches to influencing both policy-makers and practitioners directly by intervening in social problems. By the 1960s this had been transformed into researchers seeking primarily to influence policy-makers. Indeed, researchers' lofty ambitions to influence policy directly may be shaped by the shifting realities of the current policy climate. The contemporary researcher may be relatively more sanguine about their potential to influence and shape government policy, as Bloor (1997: 222) writes: 'It was pointed out by various critics that the policy community rarely sought policies from researchers: instead, research would be commissioned to confirm a preferred policy option, or perhaps to delay a necessary but inconvenient intervention.'

Bloor's historical observations are particularly useful when considering the challenges in developing practitioner research within the contemporary field, especially that of youth research. If social research has been commissioned to fulfil or develop existing policy agendas in your home organisation, there may be some real tensions in navigating the expected outcomes and actual findings generated from the study. Within the current policy landscape, the interface between contemporary practice and research has often been predicated on effectiveness, efficiency and impact; especially in developing cost-effective approaches to service delivery, identifying solutions to 'social problems' and evaluating existing social interventions. Whilst theoretically driven research continues to be funded by some of the larger research councils, much of the work within the practice arena has been oriented to assessments, evaluations and mainstreaming 'best practice' models of intervention.

Within this initial framing, Silverman (1985) considers the potential roles for sociologists and social researchers, and identifies three:

1   the scholar;
2   the state counsellor; and
3   the partisan.

These offer a helpful framework, and we now look at each in a little more detail.

## The scholar

Taking a broadly liberal position, sociologists such as Denzin (1970, drawing on Weber) argue that knowledge for knowledge's sake is the main commitment for social scientists. This means that it is a researcher's own conscience that protects the direction and basis for action for any research. Silverman (1985) highlights how such an approach resists ethical certainties, but rather mandates an individual researcher to pursue sociological activity as they see fit.

Arguably, the political implications of such an approach also uphold and reify existing power relations between powerful and powerless groups, and it is also debatable whether important ethical and value issues should be simply left to an individual researcher's judgement. There are two main issues with such an approach. The first is that the liberal scholarly approach may seem to be elitist, privileging the researcher's knowledge as 'expert'. Second, it does not consider how 'experts' and 'scientists' may be co-opted into the service of powerful interest groups.

## The state counsellor

The state counsellor model differs from that of the liberal scholar in engaging with a more 'hands-on' approach to shaping the social world. Silverman (1985) suggests that whilst Howard Becker and other similarly aligned sociologists are keen to side with the 'underdog', the state counsellor role may conversely entail siding with the powerful – the 'organisational leaders'. Silverman (1985: 183) describes the state counsellor as serving 'bureaucratic politics', and social researchers as state counsellors 'become functionaries of the state', either delivering evidence to drive policy or establishing and conceptualising new problems for policy-makers. Such a conception of the researcher follows earlier thoughts from Bulmer (1982), who suggested that social researchers might adopt an 'enlightenment' or 'engineering' model. In the former, bureaucrats may fund or commission research that fulfils their existing policy aims, and the research is thus used to legitimise their ideological ends. In the enlightenment model the researcher's role is 'to enlighten bureaucrats and not to recommend policies' (Silverman 1985: 183).

However, Silverman remains sceptical of the limits of the intellectual freedom for the researcher as state counsellor. The question here is the type of relationship social researchers should have with government agencies and, when accepting grants, what ethical tensions there might be when the research is used for social or political engineering.

## The partisan

Finally, Silverman (1985: 184) draws attention to the partisan approach: 'Unlike the scholar, the partisan does not shy away from his accountability to the world.' Becker (1967) challenged other researchers for wishing to influence elites, suggesting that the real work of the sociologist should be in actively shaping social change through a partisan sociology supporting subordinated groups. This politically engaged researcher clearly acknowledges their value base, and may actively side with the underdog (poor or young people, for example) for political ends. Wider political struggles often underpin their research endeavour in a committed action to shape the wider social world. However, again, there are tensions in this approach. Silverman suggests that within partisan Marxist research, for example, ordinary people might be situated as dupes of the system, which again positions the researcher and theorist in the powerful position of 'expert'.

Returning to the role of the social researcher, we see there is an ongoing tension for how researchers may navigate the complexities of policy and practice within professional and academic realms. Becker's call for a 'partisan' approach in social research may be highly persuasive to practitioners whose practice agenda calls for empowerment and active engagement with social justice for marginalised groups. However, Silverman's challenge to the partisan approach highlights the tensions in creating 'good research' in relation to both the research process and output. One might well ask you, as a practitioner, 'Which side are you on?' Indeed, many researchers from anti-racist and feminist traditions would clearly identify their strategic political engagement with and through the research process (Hayes and Humphries 1999; Hammersley 2001). The participatory action research (PAR) approaches that we described in Chapter 1, for example, highlight the ways in which feminists, Marxists and other researchers with clear ideological commitments to particular notions of social justice continue to champion a 'partisan' approach. As youth practitioners, the very aim of your practice may be to advocate on behalf of young people and their communities, and to uphold the values of 'social justice' in your work. Becker's argument may thus strike a chord for practitioners, especially those who work within youth work and community development fields, where 'supporting the underdog' and the agendas of empowerment and emancipatory practice are primary goals.

In exploring the role of social scientists in intervening in policy and practice, Silverman (1985) highlights that not all sociologists are in agreement with Becker's call for a partisan approach to social research. However, whilst Silverman acknowledges that not all sociologists would position themselves alongside Becker, he debunks the positivist myth of a value-free sociology (Gouldner 1962). Indeed, notions of value freedom in much social research may be questionable. For example, funders and grant-making bodies channel grants for particular routes and purposes, and such financial constraints shape the types of research, agendas and findings within the contemporary research marketplace (Silverman 1985: 179).

The action orientation of Becker's approach is thus not necessarily exclusive to social researchers trying to shape wider policy and practice matters. As Bloor (1997) notes, many contemporary social researchers are all too aware of the cross-cutting nature of accountability to funders, policy-makers, managers and other stakeholders. We can develop this idea by identifying the constellation of responsibilities in which researchers and practitioner-researchers might find themselves. Looking at the different relationships in Figure 10.1, try to identify what these might mean for your work.

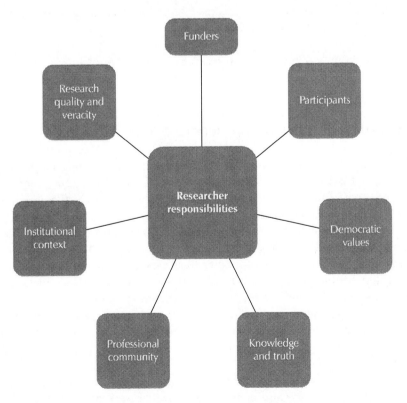

Figure 10.1 Researcher responsibilities

New researchers in the field may wish to tread carefully, perhaps preferring to tie their research aims primarily to the production of knowledge (Hammersley 1995), rather than explicitly allying their work to a partisan agenda, as this may potentially limit ability in some practice and policy contexts to defend the validity and credibility of their findings. However, in critiquing Hammersley's position, Hayes and Humphries (1999) argue that the dominant social science research culture marginalises other ways of knowing and forms of research that strive to have an active political commitment.

---

### Practice-based task 10.1  Uses for your research

In your reflective diary consider what you think your research is for.

- List all the possible uses you might find for your research.
- Look again at your list: which points are about generating new theory and ideas, or are they more about responding to existing theories?
- Which, if any, are concerned with activating 'social change' through policy and/or practice?
- In what ways might your work activate change?
- What role do you see for yourself as a social researcher: are you a scholar, a state counsellor and/or a partisan?

Write a paragraph on your response to each of these positions.

---

## Evidence-based policy and practice: a new orthodoxy

Evidence-based policy and practice has had a growing influence in such practice fields as medicine and education, emphasising as it does the need for policy- and practice-relevant research (Bulmer *et al.* 2007; Hammersley 2001). Such approaches cast research-based evidence as separate, distinct and potentially more effective than non-reflective practice knowledge. As Hammersley (2001) notes, the wider rhetoric of evidence-based practice knowledge often fails to acknowledge that 'evidence' can some-time be fallible, and does not always point to specific solutions to practice and policy dilemmas. Indeed, there are many questions about *what counts* as evidence, in *what* circumstances, and *who defines* evidence as such. Some authors have questioned the transfer of research findings in any simple linear way into practice contexts (Bulmer *et al.* 2007; Davies 2003; Hammersley 2001), particularly where evidence may be contradictory or confusing. The relationship between research, policy and practice is, inevitably, attenuated.

As the contributors have argued throughout this volume, practitioner research has become increasingly popular and significant in recent years, especially with the growing importance of evidence-based practice and the associated urge to link a *what works* approach in classrooms, welfare and health settings. As Bulmer *et al.* (2007: 87) note, '[evidence-based] policy in UK central government is not a new idea but, since 1997, we have entered a new phase between social science research and policy making'.

Rather than necessarily indicating a growing 'practice-orientated' policy, as Campbell *et al.* (2004) argue, this has often been an appropriation of *what works* models taken from medical contexts and somewhat unproblematically transferred into education and other settings. The New Labour provenance of this approach is marked and the stress on evidence-based policy emerged as a way for Blairite ministers to *modernise* and rationalise policy-making away from an (overtly) ideological basis, whilst ignoring or obscuring their own ideological motives. Whilst researchers may try to have an impact on policy and practice, Hammersley (2001) notes that the 'evidence' may not always form a neat ideological fit with policy-makers' existing agendas.

Similarly, many practitioners in the field may struggle to keep themselves up to date with systematic reviews[1] of evidence relevant to their practice settings. Both policy-makers and practitioners can also imagine they have a clear grasp of relevant issues, and therefore may choose to dismiss findings or ways of thinking that do not fit clearly with their existing views (Hammersley 2001). Indeed, Bulmer *et al.* (2007) suggest that this is a distinction drawn between *evidence-based* and *opinion-based* policy. Opinion-based work is developed through the use of selective, often non-representative studies to fulfil wider ideological ends. Whilst systematic review may support policy-makers taking the evidence-orientated *what works* approach, this is often impractical in arenas where quick responses and *hot knowledge* are required.

Let us consider two recent examples that highlight this tension and have received media coverage in the UK. Both relate to how so-called 'expert evidence' is challenged or reconfigured in the space of contemporary political and media discourse.

Drugs policy remains an especially contentious policy area as it is shaped by contrasting and conflicting moral, medical and scientific discourses. In 2009, Professor David Nutt, chairman of the UK government's Advisory Committee on the Misuse of Drugs, was sacked after presenting a research paper questioning the Labour government's stance on the classification of LSD and cannabis by suggesting current drugs policy was misguided. As one newspaper's coverage at the time stated:

> Nutt criticised [Home Secretary Jackie] Smith's use of the 'precautionary principle' to justify her decision to reclassify cannabis and said that by erring on the side of caution politicians 'distort' and 'devalue' the research evidence. 'This leads us to a position where people really don't know what the evidence is,' he said, adding that the initial decision to downgrade the classification of cannabis led to a fall in the use of the drug.
>
> (*Guardian* 2009)

We can see here how tensions between evidence and potential political realities clash in shaping contemporary drugs legislation. Whilst national governments may have committees of experts providing and reviewing research evidence to inform social policy, such relationships and the roles of the experts are fraught with difficulties and shaped by wider, instrumental and opinion-based political agendas.

A more recent example occurred when the head of the UK Office of National Statistics challenged the Coalition government ministers' (mis)use of statistics about national levels of poverty and social inequality. On 27 November 2010, the *Guardian* reported the head's concern that there had been 'serious deficiencies' in the handling of unemployment data by ministers. Meanwhile, the Trade Union Congress accused ministers of generating 'facts' to legitimise their ideologically driven cuts in welfare. This mirrors earlier work by the Government Statistics Collective (1993), which notes that policy-makers often want to 'massage' statistical findings in line with manifesto commitments and wider political agendas. As policy and practice remain shaped by questions of 'values, attitudes and ideology' (Bulmer *et al.* 2007), it might be more accurate to suggest that much of the contemporary *what works* agenda has been predicated on evidence-*informed* (rather than evidence-*based*) policy and practice.

Such examples illustrate the (perhaps inevitable) tensions and challenges to social research in directly informing policy and policy-makers. This is an interesting issue to consider in light of the prior discussion about values, political activism and social research. As we highlighted earlier, there has been a number of debates over the desirability and necessity for social researchers to aim for objectivity in social research. However, practitioner-orientated research is sometimes mistrusted in relation to ideas of neutrality and academic rigour. As Hayes and Humphries (1999: 23) argue, it is 'difficult to achieve respectability when research is viewed as "political", because a hegemony of neutral research still dominates the social science research community'.

Activist and practitioner-based approaches can directly influence local and national government policy through think-tanks, research institutes and scholarly work. Increasingly, practitioners are involved in shaping and producing research agendas and outputs. There are occasions when, arguably, partisan research has been drawn on selectively to shape and inform policy. One example is the UK Home Office's review into the sexualisation of young people (Papadopoulos 2010), which drew on a range of evidence, including previous research reports and testimonies from stakeholders such as feminist campaign groups, academics, youth professionals and media representatives to shape a response to a perceived social problem.

Social researchers may want to have a clear and active engagement with social justice principles, and they may use research to develop practice-based strategies in supporting equality work. One such example is the 'No Outsiders' project, which used participatory action research with education professionals to research and promote sexuality equality in English schools. The large project team of university-based researchers and teacher-researchers worked closely with local authorities and schools to develop gender and sexuality equality by challenging homophobic bullying and heterosexism through local education policy and practice initiatives. Teacher-researchers involved in the project located their commitment to researching school-based policy and practice interventions in light of their previous interest and activism in social movements. Their work as teacher-researchers in this project reawakened commitments to critical practice and activism (Cullen 2009).

Such a progressive research project was made possible and legitimised by its location, which bridged universities and practice settings, and the wider policy commitment to an agenda of equality and social justice through the UK Equalities Act (2010). Here, we can see how local and national policy-makers' commitments to a political cause can intersect and overlap with the development and support of potentially progressive, partisan research projects in supporting and shaping local and national policy and practice. However, it is worth noting that both the sexualisation of young people review (Papadopoulos 2010) and the No Outsiders project faced strong criticism from some sections of the media. The former was perceived as too lightweight and overly simplistic in its analysis of representation, media culture and the effects on children and young people. The latter was accused of being politically influenced and misguided, and it was portrayed (inaccurately) in the media as actively promoting homosexuality, rather than an equality agenda (Nixon 2009).

This is a somewhat murky and contentious area, with politicians and policy-makers drawing on or rejecting campaigning or traditionally neutral research project findings in light of wider political agendas. Research and practice thus remain highly political endeavours, and whilst practitioner research *can* embrace the partisan, great care is needed to establish credibility in both the research process and the research findings. Indeed, as Becker (1967: 247) argues,

> We take sides as our personal and political commitments dictate, use our theoretical and technical resources to avoid the distortions that might introduce into our work, limit our conclusions carefully, recognise the hierarchy of credibility for what it is, and field as best we can the accusations and doubts that will surely be our fate.

Becker's approach reflects the systematic, critical and self-critical enquiry that aims to contribute to advancing knowledge and practice that we advocated in Chapter 1.

## Thinking critically about politics and participation

We want to return briefly here to the contemporary public service landscape and the fashion for user participation in the fields of policy, research and practice. The participation and co-production agenda, whilst arising out of progressive politics and the practice of earlier decades, has, in recent years, evolved in parallel with the vogue for evidence-based policy and practice. Its emergence at this political juncture speaks to wider debates about neo-liberal youth and public services, increased marketisation and the positioning of service users as individualised consumers in health, education and welfare arenas, rather than reflecting earlier campaigns for empowerment and social justice for marginalised groups.

Much of the movement for greater youth participation has emerged from the policy domain. The broad participation agenda also permeated national policy, for example in a wave of early millennium UK policy. *Every Child Matters* (HM Government 2003), *Youth Matters* (HM Government 2005) and *Aiming High for Young People* (HM Treasury 2007) have all included a strong engagement with young people's rights and participation. This has two distinct roots: a children's rights approach and an extension of the communitarian call to create future 'active citizens' who are competent and fully conversant with their rights and responsibilities.

Internationally, the UN Convention on the Rights of the Child (1989) details fifty-four articles protecting children and young people's rights. It recognises that children and young people should be afforded rights protected by legislation. This legislation (Alderson 2000) links to the ongoing development of participation rights for children in a range of fields, including social research. Within these policy and research settings, children and young people have increasingly been framed as active subjects with rights, and of course this has impacted on research, policy and practice. As Heath *et al.* (2009) highlight, moves within youth policy for developing participatory approaches have been mirrored within the broader field of youth research, with an increasing drive to involve young people in research design and the conduct of social research. As earlier chapters have highlighted, research with young people, including its dissemination, is far from a value-free exercise.

Within the English youth work context, various participation audits and a burgeoning of national and local representative youth forums, emerging over the past decade or so, presuppose that these approaches to youth participation will somehow re-engage youth as a putative *at risk* group. Yet, as Bessant (2003) argues, such approaches in Australian and UK policy fail either to problematise the limits of an existing adult-centred civic domain or, typically, to call for deeper, structural forms of political engagement, such as enfranchisement. As such, an ingrained and widespread age discrimination against young people often remains unchallenged. The policy realm thus intersects and interacts with youth research agendas considering young people as a 'socially silenced' group (Alldred 1998) and represents them as active social agents and future active citizens. This broad position informs a growing movement for youth participatory research.

The moves towards young people's empowerment, particularly in youth research undertaken in policy and practice contexts, often still seemingly favours quantitative and largely positivist empiricism, rather than the kinds of collaborative, process-orientated approaches suggested by Cahill (2004, 2007) that were described in Chapter 1. Tensions emerge around managerialist agendas that permeate many contemporary practice debates. Hammersley (2001) links the evidence-based practice agenda in health and education to broader managerialist agendas. Managerialist criteria potentially position practice as predominantly a 'technical' exercise, often predicated on narrow and prescriptive notions of 'best practice'. Many educational practitioners would no doubt wish to challenge such narrow concepts of practice.

Within English youth work, trade unions, youth work scholars and practitioners have challenged technocratic and outcome-driven models of practice. In recent years, a growing 'In Defence of Youth Work' (IDYW)[2] grouping of youth workers, managers and academics has mobilised to challenge this narrow focus on providing and evidencing youth services. One of the main critiques contained in the initial IDYW open letter explaining the campaign's objectives was of an expanding technocratic practice being anathema to the process-orientated and expressive aspects of the recent historic traditions of contemporary youth work practice. The letter argued that such practice is beyond easy measurement through narrow, regimented, metric targets (Taylor 2009). Similarly, youth workers interviewed for a report raised concerns about the contemporary target-driven culture within English youth work. As Davies and Merton (2010: 26) write,

As local youth services have been required to be more accountable and conform to the disciplines of performance management, and as targets and annual plans have come to determine activities and interventions, many have expressed fears that the pursuit of targets was coming to dominate the work. Within this the risk was identified of valuing only what could be measured because measuring what is valued was difficult. In effect these workers and managers were asking: how do you count confidence, compassion, citizenship and the other outcomes on which youth workers put such emphasis?'

Such debates mirror those within wider education and social work settings, highlighting the tensions in producing evidence when becoming accountable in welfare/education services. Other critiques of such a straightforward link between evidence and practice within education settings have been framed by ideas about what constitutes valid research, notions of evidence and improvement. Indeed, research may often not be about correcting or improving practice in a linear way but rather about exploring and providing accounts of a range of social phenomena in a given context.

Davies (2003) argues that the formation and deployment of evidence within practice settings is too often a tool of neo-managerialist attempts to scrutinise and control practice through narrow definitions of practice 'quality' rather than the advancement of any critical endeavour to engage with innovative and transformative practice. She also argues that many teachers rarely have the time to participate in an ongoing critical engagement in relevant theory and research findings, nor to engage fully with their own reflexive observations. This is not to argue that research and practice cannot valuably inform one another but rather that caution should be exercised when thinking that evidence can be transferred straightforwardly into practice contexts, whether they are school, youth work or other welfare settings. Indeed, Issitt and Spence (2005) argue that youth work practice remains a rich source of material that can shape and transform policy, maintaining that the selective use of case studies, ethnographic observations, visual and virtual materials can provide a rich seam of knowledge that can offer nuanced understandings and engage more broadly with 'the social'. Such approaches may also be valuable in allowing practitioners to 'evidence' their practice.

In this light, McCulloch (2009) suggests that youth practitioners should navigate and negotiate the competing demands for the kinds of evidence, accountability and scrutiny of research and practice within managerialist agendas. Such issues have real ramifications for research and indicate the dynamics that researchers in academic, policy and practice settings have to manage in the design and implementation of any study.

## Practice-based task 10.2  Providing evidence

Consider your current work role. List the kinds of evidence of effective or successful practice that you currently provide for funders, managers and other stakeholders in your practice context.

What form does the evidence take (for example, is it quantitative or qualitative) and what is its significance in terms of the claims that you are able to make about your work?

How might you expand this body of evidence to include other forms of data that might allow you to generate other kinds of knowledge?

## How might practitioner research contribute?

Finally, we revisit Becker's question about what sociology can do for policy (and practice). As Silverman (1985: 190–191) suggests, Becker acknowledged four key roles for sociology in intervening directly with social issues:

1  'sorting out definitions of the problem' (e.g. what is the 'problem' around an issue such as teen pregnancy? How is the problem constructed? For whom is this a problem?);

2  'clarifying assumptions' (e.g. what assumptions are made about youth? What assumptions are made about youth (hetero)sexuality? How do these frame assumptions about teen pregnancy?);

3  'discovering strategic points of intervention' (e.g. through comparative work between projects and agencies, international comparisons, considering the consequences of current policy and practice interventions in sexuality education and sexual health services); and

4  'suggesting alternative moralities' (e.g. moving beyond exploring issues in administrative terms, so perhaps considering the scope to explore pleasure rather than risk in sexuality education and health work or moving beyond hetero-normative, family planning-orientated approaches within sexual health work, considering what sexual health work might be like if it were aimed primarily at regulating young men's rather than young women's sexuality, or alternatively was not orientated around a presumed heterosexuality and reproduction).

Of course, following Silverman's critique of Becker's assumptions, these interventions still potentially cast the sociologist or social scientist as a 'self-righteous' expert (Silverman 1985: 188). Yet, the role of practitioner-researcher may partially dissolve the divide between *expert* and *practitioner* knowledge and challenge accusations of elitism. Rather, in Silverman's words, the elite and elitist 'expert' knowledge of the sociologist inform the 'layman'. Thus, the practitioner-researcher role becomes actively engaged in knowledge production within and beyond the academy and practice setting.

Turning to dissemination strategies, Back (1998) argues that research is rhetorically powerful and that researchers aim to convince and persuade the reader of its veracity and worth through a range of tactics. One of the ways in which researchers may wish to make wider social commentary and social criticism is by moving beyond traditions of scholarly writing into other forms, including journalism, that may have greater impact in the policy, practice and public realms through appropriate strategies of dissemination. Of course, interacting with the media entails risks for scholars and practitioners. Media reports may misrepresent, conflate, simplify or distort findings to emphasise the 'newsworthy' aspects of a story. Writing the article oneself for a policy and practice journal may diminish these risks, but, as with all forms of dissemination, the researcher cannot control the ultimate use of their findings.

In their personal approaches to presenting their work, practitioner-researchers may move into creating a range of written and performed rhetorical outputs from research monographs, reports, magazine articles, dedicated websites, conference presentations, workshops, exhibitions, and condensed versions of their findings. All of these different outputs can be aimed at different audiences: funders, academics, policy-makers, practitioners, parents and young people. Again, such dissemination approaches can begin to dissolve the divide between the academic and public-practice realms, enabling greater opportunity for practitioner-researchers to intervene directly in social issues. As McWilliam (2004) suggests in an overview of practitioner research traditions, the notion of giving 'voice to the voiceless' has been one of the principal rationales in defending insider practitioner research.

## Practice-based task 10.3  Roles for your research

Using Becker's (1967) four key roles for social research, consider your own research project. In what ways might it contribute to the following, and to what effect:

- 'sorting out definition of the problem';
- 'clarifying assumptions';
- 'discovering strategic points of intervention'; and
- 'suggesting alternative moralities'.

Compare these with your responses to Practice-based task 10.1. Write an extract in your research journal and/or discuss with a colleague.

## Summary of main points

The key points raised in this chapter are:

- All research is political in that it has the power to shape policy and practice, or be funded or adopted for ideological purposes.

- Wider moral panics around the 'crisis' of youth have meant that youth remains an area of public, policy and research interest.
- Despite the rise of evidence-based policy and practice in education, health and welfare in recent years, there is rarely a straightforward link between research knowledge, policy interventions and practice.
- Evidence-based approaches have been linked to wider neo-managerialist agendas in public services.
- Sociologists have argued for a range of roles for researchers wishing to intervene in the policy and practice realm.
- Sociology and social science research remains an important site of intervention in constructing theory, policy and practice interventions in relation to social problems.

## Further reading

Becker's classic essay can begin to open up some of these key debates for readers:

Becker, H. (1967) 'Whose side are you on?', *Social Problems*, 14: 239–247.

Bloor also engages in an accessible way with the key debates when engaging with social problems:

Bloor, M. (1997) 'Addressing social problems through qualitative research', in D. Silverman (ed.), *Qualitative Research: Theory, method and practice*, London: Sage.

Within a youth work context, Issitt and Spence problematise the relationship between policy and practice:

Issitt, M. and Spence, J. (2005) 'Practitioner knowledge and the problem of evidence based research policy and practice', *Youth and Policy*, 88: 63–82.

## Notes

1   A systematic review is a form of literature review that attempts to produce an overview of the key, high-quality literature in areas relating to a research question or topic. Systematic reviews are often produced by various policy and research bodies on a range of topics, such as the effectiveness of drugs education, restorative youth justice and so on.
2   For more on the IDYW campaign, see: http://www.indefenceofyouthwork.org.uk/wordpress/.

## References

Alderson, P. (2000) 'Children as researchers: the effects of participation rights on research methodologies', in P. Christiansen and A. James (eds), *Research with Children: Perspectives and practice*, London: Falmer Press.

Alldred, P. (1998) 'Ethnography and discourse analysis: dilemmas in representing the voices of children', in J. Ribbens and R. Edwards (eds), *Feminist Dilemmas in Qualitative Research: Public knowledge and private lives*, London: Sage.

Armstrong, D. (2004) 'A risky business? Research, policy, governmentality and youth offending', *Youth Justice*, 4 (2): 100.

Back, L. (1998) 'Reading and writing research', in C. Seale (ed.), *Researching Society and Culture*, London: Sage.

Becker, H. (1967) 'Whose side are you on?', *Social Problems*, 14: 239–247.

Bessant, J. (2003) 'Youth participation, a new mode of government', *Policy Studies*, 24 (2/3): 87–100.

Bloor, M. (1997) 'Addressing social problems through qualitative research', in D. Silverman (ed.), *Qualitative Research: Theory, method and practice*, London: Sage.

Bulmer, M. (1982*) The Uses of Social Research*, London: Allen and Unwin.

Bulmer, M., Coates, E. and Dominian, L. (2007) 'Evidence-based policymaking', in H. Boches and S. Duncan (eds), *Making Policy in Theory and Practice*, Bristol: Policy Press.

Cahill, C. (2004) 'Defying gravity? Raising consciousness through collective research', *Children's Geographies*, 2 (2): 273–286.

Cahill, C. (2007) 'Doing research with young people: participatory research and the rituals of collective work', *Children's Geographies*, 5 (3): 297–312.

Campbell, A., McNamara, O. and Gilroy, P. (2004) *Practitioner Research and Professional Development in Education*, London: Paul Chapman.

Cullen, F. (2009) 'Seeking a queer(ying) pedagogic praxis: adventures in the classroom and participatory action research', in R. DePalma and E. Atkinson (eds), *Interrogating Heteronormativity: Researching sexualities equalities in school*, Stoke on Trent: Trentham Press.

Davies, B. (2003) 'Death to critique and dissent? The policies and practices of new managerialism and "evidence-based practice"', *Gender and Education*, 15 (1): 91–103.

Davies, B. and Merton, B. (2010) *Straws in the Wind: The state of youth work practice in a changing policy environment (Phase 2)*, DeMontford University. http://www.dmu.ac.uk/Images/Straws%20in%20the%20Wind%20-%20Final%20Report%20-%20October%202010_tcm6-67206.pdf (accessed 20/11/2010).

Denzin, N.K. (1970) *The Research Act in Sociology*, London: Butterworth.

Gouldner, A. (1962) 'Anti minotaurs', *Social Problems*, 9: 199–213.

*Government Statisticians' Collective* (1993) 'How official statistics are produced: views from the inside', in M. Hammersley (ed.), *Social Research, Philosophy, Politics and Practice*, London: Sage.

Griffin, C. (1993) *Representations of Youth: The study of youth and adolescence in Britain and America*, Cambridge: Polity Press.

*Guardian* (2009) 'Alcohol worse than ecstasy – drugs chief.' http://www.guardian.co.uk/politics/2009/oct/29/nutt-drugs-policy-reform-call (accessed 18/11/2010).

*Guardian* (2010) 'Welfare ministers rebuked over poor data,' 27 November: 26.

Hammersley, M. (1995) *The Politics of Social Research*, London: Sage.

Hammersley, M. (2001) 'Some questions about evidence-based practice in education', paper presented to the British Educational Research Association, University of Leeds, 13–15 September.

Hayes, D. and Humphries, B. (1999) 'Negotiating contentious research topics', in B. Broad (ed.), *The Politics of Social Work Research and Evaluation*, Birmingham: Venture Press.

Heath, S., Brooks, R., Cleaver, E. and Ireland, E. (2009) *Researching Young People's Lives*, London: Sage.

HM Government (2003) *Every Child Matters: Change for children*, London: Department for Education and Skills.

HM Government (2005) *Youth Matters*, London, Department for Education and Skills.

HM Treasury (2007) *Aiming High for Young People: A ten-year strategy for positive activities*, London: HM Treasury/Department for Children, Schools and Families.

Issitt, M. and Spence, J. (2005) 'Practitioner knowledge and the problem of evidence based research policy and practice', *Youth and Policy*, 88: 63–82.

Jeffs, T. and Smith, M.K. (1999) 'The problem of "youth" for youth work', *Youth and Policy*, 62: 45–66.

Jenks, C. (2005) *Childhood*, 2nd edn, London: Routledge.

Jones, G. (2009) *Youth*, Cambridge: Polity Press.

McCulloch, K. (2009) 'Ethics, accountability and the shaping of youth work practice', in R. Harrison, C. Benjamin, S. Curran and R. Hunter (eds), *Leading Work with Young People*, London: Sage/Open University Press.

McWilliam, E. (2004) 'W(h)ither practitioner research?', *Australian Educational Researcher*, 31 (2): 113–126.

Middleton, E. (2006) 'Youth participation in the UK: bureaucratic disaster or triumph of child rights?', *Children, Youth and Environment*, 16 (2): 180–190.

Nixon, D. (2009) '"Vanilla" strategies: compromise or collusion?', in R. DePalma and E. Atkinson (eds), *Interrogating Heteronormativity: Researching sexualities equalities in school*, Stoke on Trent: Trentham Press.

Papadopoulos, L. (2010) *Sexualisation of Young People: A review*, UK Home Office. http://webarchive.nationalarchives.gov.uk/+/http://www.homeoffice.gov.uk/documents/s exualisation-of-young-people.pdf (accessed 25/11/2010).

Silverman, D. (1985) *Qualitative Methodology and Sociology*, London: Gower.

Smith, M.K. (2004) 'Extended schooling: some issues for informal and community education', in *The Encyclopedia of Informal Education*. http://www.infed.org/schooling/ extended_schooling.htm (accessed 19/09/2008).

Taylor, T. (2009) 'In defence of youth work', open letter. http://indefenceofyouthwork. wordpress.com/2009/03/11/the-open-letter-in-defence-of-youth-work/ (accessed 10/10/ 2010).

Watts, G. (2002) 'Connexions: the role of a personal advisor in schools', *Pastoral Care in Education*, 19 (4): 16–20.

West, A. (1999) 'Young people as researchers: ethical issues in participatory research', in S. Banks (ed.), *Ethical Issues in Youth Work*, London: Routledge.

## Useful websites

The following websites provide links, downloadable tools and case studies on participatory youth approaches in youth practice and research contexts.

Australian Clearing House on Youth Studies (participation page – links to readings and resources): http://www.acys.info/resources/topics/participation

FreeChild project (US-based website that provides tools for young people and adults who engage children and youth in social change): http://www.freechild.org/index.htm

No Outsiders research project: www.nooutsiders.sunderland.ac.uk

Young Researchers Network (UK): http://www.nya.org.uk/integrated-youth-support-services/ young-researcher-network

# Index